NURSES' PERCEPTIONS OF SPIRITUAL CARE

For my grandmother Jean and my parents Jim and Margaret Waugh

As you ought not to attempt to cure the eyes without the head, or the head
without the body, so neither ought you to attempt to cure the body without
the soul... for the part can never be well unless the whole is well.
(Plato in Sims 1987, p.65)

Spiritual is what is human to man.
(Frankl in Granstrom 1985, p.41)

Nurses' Perceptions of Spiritual Care

LINDA A. ROSS (Nee Waugh)
BA Nursing, RGN, PhD

Avebury

Aldershot • Brookfield USA • Hong Kong • Singapore • Sydney

Published by
Avebury
Ashgate Publishing Ltd
Gower House
Croft Road
Aldershot
Hants GU11 3HR
England

Ashgate Publishing Company
Old Post Road
Brookfield
Vermont 05036
USA

British Library Cataloguing in Publication Data

Ross, Linda
    Nurses' perceptions of spiritual care. - (Developments in nursing and health care)
    1. Nursing - Religious aspects
    I. Title
    610.7'3'069

Library of Congress Catalog Card Number: 97-70635

ISBN 1 85972 618 6

Printed and bound by Athenaeum Press, Ltd., Gateshead, Tyne & Wear.

Contents

Figures and tables

ix

Acknowledgements

Numerous people assisted with this study. Unfortunately, it is not possible to name them individually. Some, however, require special mention.

First, I would like to thank Queen Margaret College, Edinburgh for providing the opportunity, funding and resources which enabled this study to be conducted. I would also like to express my gratitude to my colleagues in various departments in the College, especially those in the Department of Health and Nursing, for their support in so many ways. Furthermore I am grateful to the staff of Queen Margaret College library for their help in tracing many obscure references.

I am indebted to my director of studies, Dr L Hockey (Honorary Reader, Visiting Professor) and supervisors, Rev Dr D Lyall (Senior Lecturer, Department of Christian Ethics and Practical Theology, University of Edinburgh) and Ms E Dove (retired Co-ordinator of the Resource Unit for Motor Disorder, Queen Margaret College) for their untiring guidance, advice, support and patience throughout the many stages of this project.

Special thanks are due to the managerial staff of the various Health Boards and to the nurses who participated in the study. Without them this research project would not have been possible.

I also owe my gratitude to Mark for his encouragement, patience and for the many hours he invested transcribing interviews, assisting with graphics and proof reading numerous drafts of chapters. Finally my parents, Margaret and Jim Waugh require special mention. Not only did they support me morally and financially but also gave selflessly of their time. They assisted in the coding of questionnaires as well as helping me in so many practical ways, thereby enabling the study to reach a timely conclusion.

Preface

There is evidence of increasing interest and awareness of the contribution of the spiritual dimension to health, recovery and well-being. Conferences, study days and workshops addressing the topic are being offered by health care professionals in response to demand from other health care professionals. Recent years have also seen an increase in the number of nursing and medical journal articles stressing the importance of this aspect of care and questioning how it might be addressed. The nursing literature considers spiritual care part of the nurse's role but guidelines for its practice are lacking. Research on spiritual care, particularly of British origin, is very much in its infancy and little is known about how British nurses perceive their role in this.

This book reports a study, believed to be the first of its kind in Britain, which sought to ascertain how nurses, working in care of the elderly hospitals in Scotland, perceived spiritual need and spiritual care and professed to have given this care in practice. Factors which appeared to influence the spiritual care nurses gave were also explored. Given the descriptive nature of the study its prescriptive function is limited highlighting the need for further research in this important area of patient care.

Abbreviations, assumptions and terms

Abbreviations

AACN	American Association of Colleges of Nursing
ICN	International Council of Nurses
NHS	National Health Service
NBS	National Board for Nursing, Midwifery and Health Visiting for Scotland
NANDA	North American Nursing Diagnosis Association
RGN	Registered General Nurse
SPSS	Statistical Package for the Social Sciences
SRN	State Registered Nurse
UKCC	United Kingdom Central Council for Nursing, Midwifery and Health Visiting

Assumptions

For the purpose of this study the following assumptions are made:

1 The spiritual dimension is an innate element of every human being, regardless of the presence or absence of religious beliefs and practices. As such, all human beings have spiritual needs.

2 An optimum state of health, well-being and quality of life is valued by and striven for by all human beings.

Terms

Statements relating to nurses' perceptions of spiritual need and spiritual care and how they gave this care refer to their *reports* about each.

The terms 'tendency to' and 'influence' are used in the discussion of the study results, in a non-statistical sense.

Quotations from Scripture are taken from the Good News Bible.

Clergy	The recognised spiritual representative of any denomination, e.g., minister, rabbi.
Conservatism	A strong religious conviction of a fundamentalist nature.
Full-time	Any nurse working 30 hours or more per week.
General hospital	Any hospital containing a care of the elderly ward and one or more of the following as classified by Chaplin (1989): 'general / mixed acute / infectious diseases / chest / medicine / surgery / paediatric / orthopaedic / ENT / obstetric / maternity'.
Geriatric hospital	Any hospital containing one or more of the following as hospital classified by Chaplin (1989):'geriatric / long stay / assessment / continuing care / rehabilitation'.
God	Higher power as defined by the individual.
Indirect verbal communication	Conveyance of a message through the emphasis placed on certain words and the tone of voice.
Non-psychiatric care of the elderly ward	Any care of the elderly ward classified as such by the nurse managers of the hospitals approached but excluding those classified by Chaplin (1989) as: 'psychiatry / mental illness / mental handicap / psycho-geriatric'.
Non-varied	Chronic geriatric ward only, e.g., long term care or acute geriatric ward only, e.g., geriatric medicine.
Religious affiliation	Label adopted by an individual to signify their belief system.

Spiritual care	Making arrangements for the provision of patients' spiritual needs.
Spiritual dimension	That element within the individual from which originates: meaning, purpose and fulfilment in life; a will to live; belief and faith in self, others and God and which is essential to the attainment of an optimum state of health, well-being or quality of life.
Spiritual distress	The state resulting when an individual is deprived of having their spiritual needs fulfilled.
Spiritual need	A lack of any or all of the following which are required to produce spiritual well-being: meaning, purpose and fulfilment in life; the will to live; belief and faith in self, others and God.
Spiritual well-being	The overall state of spiritual health which is evidenced by the presence of: meaning, purpose and fulfilment in life; the will to live; belief and faith in self, others and God.
Varied ward	Combination of chronic and acute care, e.g., long term care and geriatric medicine.

Part One
A REVIEW OF THE LITERATURE

1 Introduction

The author's interest in the subject of spiritual care was stimulated following an encounter with a terminally ill patient. Having been asked if she would like a passage read to her from the Bible lying on her locker, the change in this woman's expression was remarkable. Instead of lying sleeping, or staring blankly into space, her eyes widened, she strained to raise her head, smiled and attempted to speak for the first time in several months. Later, just before she died, she expressed how much this, together with prayer, had meant to her. She said 'I love you and thank you'. She had a spiritual need which she required to have met.

This profound and moving experience suggested to the author that the spiritual dimension could have a considerable influence on a patient's quality of life while in hospital. In this instance, however, trained staff appeared to allow other tasks, such as tidying the linen cupboard, to assume priority over spiritual care.

It was with the desire to discover more, from the literature, about the relationship between the spiritual dimension, health and quality of life that an under-graduate research proposal was designed (Waugh, 1986). The proposal formed the basis for this study which aims to: 1) ascertain how a sample of nurses, working in Scotland, perceive spiritual need and spiritual care and profess to give it in practice 2) identify factors appearing to influence spiritual care.

In Part 1 the relevant literature on spiritual care is reviewed. First, evidence is presented for the influence of the spiritual dimension on health, well-being and quality of life (Chapter 2). Second, spiritual care is presented as part of the nurse's role (Chapters 3 and 4). However, it is shown that guidelines for its practice are currently lacking and that patients' spiritual needs may not be well attended to (Chapter 5).

A conceptual framework for giving spiritual care, based on the nursing process, is suggested in Part 2, but has not yet been tested.

Part 3 gives an overview of the study outlining the research questions and the blend of quantitative and qualitative approaches adopted to address them. A more detailed account of the quantitative and qualitative approaches is given in Parts 4 and 5 respectively and within each relevant findings are presented and discussed.

In the final Part (Part 6) conclusions are drawn from the findings, their implications are discussed and suggestions for practice and further research are proposed.

2 The influence of the spiritual dimension on health, well-being and quality of life

It is the purpose of this chapter to describe and define the main concepts used throughout the text, e.g., the 'spiritual dimension' and 'spiritual need'. It is then illustrated how vital these concepts are to the attainment of an optimum state of health, well-being and quality of life which are goals generally striven for by all human beings. The experiences of illness and hospitalisation are then presented as potential crises which can result in spiritual distress thereby preventing or diminishing the individual's ability to achieve these supreme goals.

The inseparability of the concepts of health, well-being and quality of life

First, it is necessary to look at definitions of health, well-being and quality of life and to illustrate that all three terms are inseparably linked.

Quality of life has been defined by Dalkey and Rourke (in Ferrans and Powers, 1985, pp.15-16) as:

> a person's sense of well-being, his satisfaction or dissatisfaction with life, or his happiness or unhappiness.

The World Health Organisation (WHO) (in Kratz, 1979, p.22) defines health as:

> a complete state of physical, mental and social well-being, and not merely the absence of disease or infirmity.

From the above two definitions, it can be seen that both 'quality of life' and 'health' can be equated with 'well-being', indicating that all three terms are inseparably linked.

Furthermore, quality of life is defined in terms of the individual's satisfaction with life. Satisfaction has been defined by Campbell et al. (in Ferrans and Powers, 1985, p.17) as:

the perceived discrepancy between what is aspired to and what is achieved.

and has increasingly been recognised as the most important indicator of quality of life. Quality of life has been described as 'the satisfaction of needs' (Ferrans and Powers, 1985, p.17). It could be argued, therefore, that the level of quality of life and hence the state of health or well-being (having established the inseparability of these terms) attained by an individual, will be determined by the degree to which their physical, mental and social needs are met with total fulfilment and with total deprivation (if such states actually exist) occupying opposite ends of the quality of life continuum (Figure 1.1).

Similarly, the literature reviewed frequently acknowledged the human being as a biopsychosocial being, all three dimensions being inter-related and constantly interacting, change in any one subsequently affecting all others. Brewer (1979) is one such theorist who considers the three dimensions to be directly related to the quality of life experienced in every day living.

Tubesing (1979), however, stresses the importance of realising that the human being is greater than the sum of his/her individual parts and should thus be considered in his/her entirety. This holistic concept of humankind is by no means a new invention. It can be traced back to the Indo-European root 'kailo' meaning whole or intact. Over several thousand years a number of other words, such as holy, heal, health and whole were derived from it (Hitchens 1988).

Important as it is to view a person as a whole biopsychosocial being, this still presents an inadequate and incomplete profile by ignoring a further essential element - the spiritual dimension. Its importance is aptly stated by De Lourdes (in Thorson and Cook, 1980, p.139):

Spiritual well-being supersedes all other values. It is the supreme affirmation of life. To ignore or attempt to separate the need to fulfil the spiritual well-being of a man from attempts to satisfy his physical, material and social needs is to fail to understand the meaning of man.

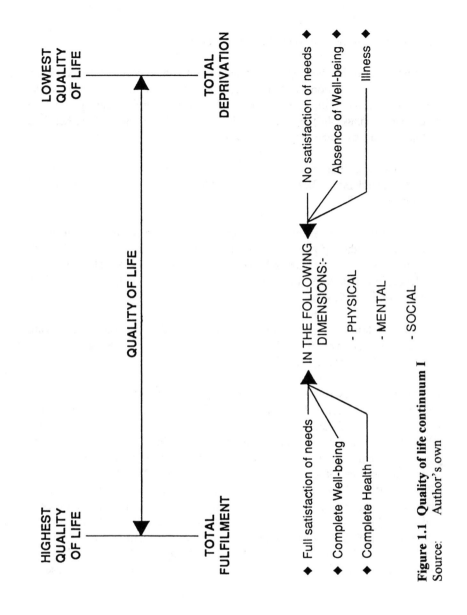

Figure 1.1 Quality of life continuum I
Source: Author's own

Description and definition of the spiritual dimension

Spiritual integrity has been suggested as a basic human need (O'Brien, 1982). According to the dictionary (MacDonald, 1972) the 'spirit' is defined as: the vital principle; the soul; a breath of wind; essence; chief quality; that which gives real meaning. In the literature, the spiritual dimension is described in a multiplicity of ways including the following:

1   The part which strives for meaning and purpose in existence (Dickinson, 1975, Henderson, 1973, Piepgras, 1973, Travelbee, 1971, Tillich in Hitchens, 1988).

2   The part which strives for transcendence beyond the here and now in search of some higher power or God (however defined by the individual) /something greater than self (Fish and Shelly, 1978, Henderson in Henderson and Nite, 1978, Martin and Carlson, 1988, O'Brien, 1982, Stallwood, 1975).

3   That which inspires, motivates and hopes, directing the individual toward the values of love, truth, beauty, trust and creativity (Dickinson, 1975, O'Brien, 1982, Stoll, 1979, Travelbee, 1971).

From the above descriptions, the spiritual dimension would appear to be a very complex phenomenon. It has been regarded as the central 'artery' which permeates, energises and enlivens all of the other dimensions of human kind (Brewer, 1979) and around which all values, thoughts, decisions, behaviours, experiences and ultimate concerns are centred. As such it has been described as the mainstream of life (Dickinson, 1975, Stoll, 1979, Yura and Walsh, 1982) and it has been suggested that without spiritual well-being these other dimensions of man can never function or be developed to their fullest capacity and hence the highest quality of life is unattainable. Brewer (1979) is but one author who depicts the spiritual dimension in a model (Figure 1.2).

Brewer recognises four aspects of the human being, all of which are involved in day to day living and contribute to the quality of life experienced. These are the:

1   Psychical, or 'I - me' relationship. This is the highest form of consciousness known, where there exists an awareness of the self through which all things are experienced.

2   Physical, or 'I - it', 'I - my body', relationship. This involves the individual's relationship with the environment.

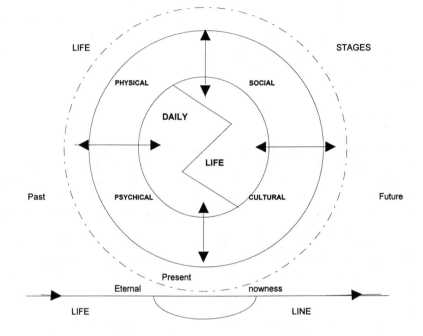

Figure 1.2 Model of spiritual well-being

Source: Reproduced by kind permission of University Press of America
           from Brewer, D.C. (1979), 'Life Stages and Spiritual Well-being',
           in Moberg, D.O. (ed.), *Spiritual Well-being: Sociological
           Perspectives*, University Press of America: Washington

3 Social, or 'I - you', 'I - them' relationship. This refers to the individual's
   relationship with other fellow human beings, whether as individuals or
   groups.

4. Cultural or the attitudes, norms, expectations, values and beliefs (in this study the 'cultural' is referred to under the 'social').

The interaction of these aspects in daily life is dynamic and constantly changing, all aspects influencing the various life stages, i.e., past, present and future (outer dotted circle), as viewed at any one point on the 'Life line' (x - axis on diagram).

However, the point to note is the way in which the spiritual dimension pervades all other dimensions and life stages, allowing for transcendence beyond the ordinary to the extra-ordinary and mystical, thus adding a new dimension and quality to daily living.

From the definitions and descriptions of the spiritual dimension given above it would appear that it is a dual concept consisting of both vertical and horizontal elements as follows.

Vertical element

The vertical element could be considered to encompass the transcendental, i.e., the individual's relationship with God. Although religion with its respective rituals and customs may be one vehicle through which some people experience this relationship, it should not be assumed that the practice of religion by an individual indicates the existence of this relationship. Similarly, the absence of religious practice does not negate it.

For others, such as humanists, the transcendent need not take the form of relationship with/awareness of God but rather may constitute the individual's value system which forms the focus of their life. As Stoll states (in Rinear and Buys, 1985, p. 867):

> man is incurably religious...what varies among men is what they are religious about. Whatever a person thinks to be the highest value in life can be regarded as his god, the focus and purpose of his time and life.

Horizontal element

The horizontal element could be thought of as an outworking of the vertical in the individual's life-style and relationships with self, others and environment.

In summary, the spiritual dimension is a universal aspect of the human being which extends beyond the narrow bounds of religion, stimulating the individual to transcend the realms of the material, psychosocial and ordinariness of every day life, in search of ultimate meaning, purpose and fulfilment in their existence (Kiening, 1978, Zentner et al., 1979).

10

The definition which probably best captures and summarises the spiritual dimension is that of Renetzky (1979) who defines it in terms of its three component parts namely:

1 The 'power within man' giving 'meaning, purpose and fulfilment' (MPF) to life, suffering and death.

2 The individual's 'will to live'.

3 The individual's belief and faith in self, others and a 'power beyond self' or God.

Given the elements in Renetzky's definition, together with the fact that the spiritual dimension supersedes all other dimensions, for the purpose of this study it can be defined as:

that element within man, from which originates: meaning, purpose and fulfilment in life; a will to live; belief and faith in self, others and God, and which is essential to the attainment of an optimum state of well-being, health or quality of life.

Having described and defined the spiritual dimension, attention now focuses on spiritual need.

Description and definition of spiritual need

Spiritual need has been defined in a number of ways by different authors. According to Stallwood and Stoll (in Stoll, 1983, p.15) it is:

any factor necessary to establish and/or maintain a person's dynamic personal relationship with God (as defined by that individual) and out of that relationship to experience forgiveness, love, hope, trust and meaning and purpose in life.

Central to the above definition is the individual's relationship with God (as defined by that individual) out of which is experienced:

1 Meaning and purpose in life.
2 Hope.
3 Trust and faith in someone outwith self.
4 Love - unconditional from self, others and God.

5   Forgiveness - from self, others and God.

Spiritual needs included in the study by Highfield and Cason (1983) were based on Clinebell's 'religious-existential framework' and included the need:

1   For meaning and purpose.
2   To receive love.
3   To give love.
4   For hope and creativity.

The authors also contend that the above needs are met through the individual's relationship with God, although interpretation of this is left to the reader.
   In a similar vein Fish and Shelly (1978) define spiritual need as the need for:

1   Meaning and purpose.
2   Love and relatedness.
3   Forgiveness.

Although they acknowledge that these needs can be met in part from other sources, they contest that they can only be fully met through a dynamic, personal relationship with God.
   Common to all these definitions of spiritual need is the vertical element of spirituality, i.e., the individual's relationship with/awareness of God which works out in the horizontal, i.e., in relationships with self, others and the environment enabling the individual to experience creativity, love, forgiveness, relatedness, trust, faith and to find hope, meaning and purpose in their existence.
   These various spiritual needs can be placed under the umbrella of the spiritual dimension definition as illustrated in Figure 1.3.
   Having identified the various facets of spiritual need from definitions given in the literature, it was considered necessary to develop an operational definition of the term for the purpose of this study.
   According to Maslow (in DiCaprio, 1974), the meeting of 'lower' or 'deficit' needs (e.g., physiological/safety needs) is essential for survival, but to consider these needs alone is insufficient.
   He holds that gratification of less obvious and more fragile 'growth' needs, e.g., the need to 'know and understand' and 'find meaning in life' (clearly spiritual needs) is just as important.
   In Maslow's opinion, the fulfilment of these needs is essential for the attainment of self actualisation, which he regards as the force for growth, without which one cannot fulfil:

ones individual nature in all its aspects, being what one can be (Maslow in DiCaprio 1974, p241).

It is through this self-actualisation process, or state of 'becoming', that ultimate fulfilment and satisfaction are experienced (Maslow, 1970) and total healthy functioning achieved.

Aspects of the spiritual dimension from the definition	meaning, purpose & fulfilment	will to live	belief and faith in self, others and God
Spiritual needs identified in literature	- meaning and purpose - creativity (this aspect could arguably fit anywhere. It has been placed here for ease on the premise that being creative, whether expressed through art, music, poetry or relationships, essentially embodies life with meaning).	-hope is equated with will to live later in discussion)	- relationship with /aware-ness of God - love - forgiveness - relatedness - trust - faith

Figure 1.3 Comparison of the spiritual needs identified in the literature with the three aspects of the spiritual dimension definition
Source: Author's own

Maslow thus regards the tension produced from growth needs (spiritual needs) as positive. Selye (1980) similarly considers 'good' or 'eustressing' stressors as essential motivators enabling the individual to experience achievement and fulfilment. Given Maslow's definition of 'need' as:

a deficit state, a lack of something that is required (in DiCaprio, 1974, p. 422)

a 'growth need' could be defined as:

a lack of something that produces growth.

If a spiritual need is a growth need, it could be defined thus:

a lack of any or all of the following required to produce growth: meaning, purpose and fulfilment in life; the will to live; belief and faith in self, others and God.

Maslow postulates that if need deprivation is experienced some form of illness results. Spiritual distress could, therefore, be defined as:

the state resulting when an individual is deprived of having their spiritual needs fulfilled.

Just as it is possible to experience spiritual distress, it is also possible to experience the opposite state, i.e., spiritual well-being. This can, therefore, be defined as:

the overall state of spiritual health which is evidenced by the presence of: MPF in life; the will to live; belief and faith in self, others and God.

It is evident, therefore, that well-being, health and quality of life are essentially dependent on the extent to which spiritual needs are satisfied.

Although Maslow (in DiCaprio, 1974) holds that deficit needs should be met to a certain extent before growth needs can be considered, he also acknowledges that this is not always necessary. Thus, although biopsychosocial well-being is dependent on the degree of spiritual well-being (e.g., the effect of loss of hope), the latter can be attained and self-actualisation continue, despite the degree of biopsychosocial well-being (e.g., the person who suffers incredible physical torture rather than give up their faith).

Having described and defined spiritual need, it would appear that for the attainment of an optimum state of health, quality of life or well-being, spiritual needs require to be met.

Evidence for the influence of the spiritual dimension on health, well-being and quality of life

So far, the influence of the spiritual dimension on health, well-being and quality of life has merely been argued and is summarised by Jourard when he states:

> hope, purpose, meaning and direction in life produce and maintain wellness...whereas demoralisation by events and conditions of daily existence help people become ill (in Hitchens, 1988, p.17).

Support for the influence of the spiritual dimension on health, well-being and quality of life is presented by considering each component of the spiritual dimension in turn, as available in the literature.

Meaning and purpose

Taking the first component, according to Yura and Walsh (1982, p. 90):

> the greatest task of human kind is to determine the meaning of life.

Stoll states:

> It has been said that man needs reasons for living and if there are none he begins to die (in Rinear and Buys, 1985, p. 867).

Furthermore, Frankl and Travelbee (in Dickinson, 1975), together with many other authors, regard this as a universal trait which is essential to life itself (Autton, 1980, Colliton, 1981).

Burnard (1989) and Frankl (1959) assert that, when there is an inability to invest life with meaning, spiritual distress is the outcome characterised by feelings of emptiness and despair.

The necessity of meaning in life is similarly reflected in a number of psychological theories. McClymont et al. (1976) report how both Jung and Peck postulate respectively that meaning is necessary for the maintenance of ego integrity and for the prevention of restlessness and deterioration in old age.

Furthermore, a number of research studies highlight the importance of meaning in life for health and well-being.

Simsen (1985) found that medical and surgical patients demonstrated a need to find meaning in their illness and hospitalisation. Although based on a small sample of 45 patients in a specific area in England, the study indicates that, within the sample, search for meaning was a significant experience for these patients. This was one of the few British studies addressing spirituality.

Kobasa (in Martin and Carlson, 1988) reported fewer negative stress symptoms in individuals who were committed to and found meaning in their work. Detailed information about the method used was, however, not available and hence validity and reliability of the results were not clear. Also Antonovsky (1979) and Frankl (1959), in their observations of holocaust victims, reported survival, minimal psychological damage and even strengthening of character in those who had managed to maintain a sense of meaning and purpose in their lives throughout their ordeal.

Renetzky (1979) sought to discover the relationship between MPF, as measured by the 'Personal well-being x-ray' (Figure 1.4), and spiritual well-being, as measured by the extent of the religious role within an individual, which as already stated can act as an avenue through which the spiritual is expressed. As human life primarily consists of a number of inter-related roles, it is to be expected that MPF will normally be achieved through these roles.

Given that the percentage of MPF obtained from a role is not necessarily related to the length of time or amount of energy expended on it (e.g., it is possible to spend a long time in a role but achieve little MPF) then it is possible for there to exist a degree of emptiness or 'void' within an individual (as previously highlighted by Burnard 1989 and Frankl 1959). If the attainment of MPF is vital to life, then a large amount of 'void' is detrimental to the individual.

Out of a 1,000 cases in his clinical experience (he does not detail the selection of the sample) Renetzky found that as MPF increased so did the role of religion and the degree of healthy self love (as measured by 'the self wheel', a tool developed using a 1-10 scale). A decrease in the 'void' equated with an increase in spiritual well-being.

The findings of this single study conducted in the USA cannot be generalised. However, it supports the supposition that, as MPF increases, so does the level of spiritual well-being and consequently quality of life and health.

To summarise this section, it would appear that the quest for MPF in life is fundamental to the attainment of an optimum state of health, well-being and quality of life.

Will to live

The second component of the spiritual dimension is the individual's 'will to live', the importance of which is illustrated in the following quotation from Proverbs 18:14 (Holy Bible):

Your will to live can sustain you when you are sick, but if you lose it, your hope is gone.

MALE ROLES*	Meaning	Purpose	Fulfilment
1 Husband			
Divorcee			
Widower			
Sweetheart			
2 Father			
3 Job (breadwinner)			
4 Son			
5 Brother			
6 Uncle			
7 Grandfather			
8 Self			
9 Friend			
10 Religion			
11 Student			
12 Maintenance man			
13 Others			
14 Void			
	100%	100%	100%

* Corresponding female roles

1 Wife	4 Daughter	10 Religion
Divorced	5 Sister	11 Student
Widow	6 Aunt	12 Home maker
Sweetheart	7 Grandmother	13 Others
2 Mother	8 Self	14 Void
3 Job (breadwinner)	9 Friend	

The client is asked to identify the particular roles which make up his/her life, and to assign to each role the percentage of meaning, purpose and fulfilment derived from each (cannot exceed 100%). From this the degree of void and MPF as a whole can be indicated, thus giving some idea of the quality of life experienced by the individual.

Figure 1.4 The measurement of personal well-being using the personal well-being x-ray

Source: Reproduced by kind permission of University Press of America from Renetzky (1979), 'The Fourth Dimension: Applications to the Social Services', in Moberg, D.O. (ed.), *Spiritual Well-being: Sociological Perspectives*, University Press of America: Washington.

It can also be seen from this quotation that the 'will to live' and 'hope' are inseparably linked, the latter having been defined as:

to desire with belief in the possibility of fulfilment (Kirkpatrick, 1983, p. 604).

As such, hope has been regarded as a major motivator of behaviour, acting as a powerful life force, producing vitality and liveliness in life (Dubree and Vogelpohl ,1980). Widespread documentation gives evidence of the fact that without it, death can result. For instance, both animal and human studies show that prolonged and repeated encounters with situations, which although not life threatening are unavoidable, and in which the outcome is independent of all voluntary responding, produce helplessness/hopelessness. The end product of this is frequently death. Such instances include voodoo death and concentration camp experiences, as cited by Cannon and Burrel (in Seligman, 1974), Bettleheim (in Seligman, 1974) and Frankl (1963) respectively. Furthermore, although a causal link is difficult to identify, Blenkner (1967) noted higher mortality rates in elderly people who had been involuntarily institutionalised. It is because of its often drastic effects that helplessness/hopelessness has been appropriately termed as 'passive suicide' (Limandri and Boyle, 1978, p.79).

The importance of hope to life can be seen, not only in death caused by its absence, but also in healing produced by its abundance. These two states demonstrate the extremes of the hope-hopeless/helplessness continuum :-

Continuum

Hope	Hopelessness/ helplessness
can result in physical healing and well-being	can result in death

Evidence for the positive effects of hope can be seen in clinicians' observations of clients over a number of years. For instance both Renetzky (1979) and Swaim (1962) reported that the greater the will to live, the greater the chance their clients had of overcoming illness.

A different type of evidence which reports non-verifiable events, illustrates the positive effects of hope. For example Gardner (1983) and Tari (1978) document numerous instances of miraculous events e.g healing of the deaf and blind, raising of the dead where hope and also faith in God were central. These instances are hardly surprising if, as McGee (1984) states, the degree of

18

hope is related to the perception of the individual with regard to what is desired as probable. The bigger one's concept of God, the more things become possible and obtainable.

It is in recognition of the importance of hope that Dominian (1983), a psychiatrist, acknowledged that medical prognosis cannot be established on the basis of scientific data alone, but must be made in conjunction with the hope displayed by the patient.

It would appear, therefore, that hope or a will to live is vital to life itself.

Belief and faith in self, others and God

The third component of the spiritual dimension is that of 'belief and faith in self, others and God'.

In over 30 years working as a sociologist, Renetzky (1979) reported his observation that, as an individual's belief in self and others increases, so does the will to live. Furthermore this latter aspect, together with MPF and spiritual well-being, were increased to a significantly greater degree when there existed, in addition, belief in God. Consequently there was virtual extinguishing of the 'void'.

Renetzky (1979) reported that the factor above all else which appeared to influence the individual's spiritual well-being, and hence their state of health and quality of life, was belief in God.

Just as belief is important in the attainment of spiritual well-being, health and a quality of life, this is also true of faith.

It is important to distinguish between these two concepts, in that it is possible to have belief without faith, yet impossible to have faith without belief, e.g., one can believe that people exist, yet fail to have faith in them, however one cannot have faith in them without first believing that they exist. Faith then, can be viewed as belief in action, the latter having become personal and meaningful.

Renetzky (1979) reported that spiritual well-being was greatest in those who had invested belief and faith in God. Not only were they able to cope more calmly throughout difficulties, but they also possessed a higher MPF and will to live and a lower 'void' than those who had no faith in God. Furthermore, as the individual's concept of God became bigger, so these attributes increased even further in degree, as did their quality of life.

Other studies have indicated the influence of belief and faith on health. O'Brien (1982) noted that patients who possessed a positive religious perspective on life adapted more readily to the stress of haemodialysis. Martin and Carlson (1988) reported the findings of two studies by Carlson et al. (1986) and Byrd (1984) which indicated the therapeutic effect of faith in reducing anger, anxiety, pulmonary oedema and need for antibiotic therapy, and intubation respectively. However, Martin and Carlson (1988) question these findings given the biased samples used and absence of tests to determine statistical significance.

Although further research is indicated to test these observations, it would appear that the optimum state of health, quality of life or well-being, can only be attained when MPF in life, a will to live and belief and faith in self, others and God exist (Figure 1.5).

Illness and hospitalisation as spiritual encounters

The spiritual dimension has been discussed with reference to healthy people who achieve need gratification, first by being motivated, and then by initiating action. There are however, a number of forces which can interfere with the ability of an individual to seek need fulfilment. Illness and/or hospitalisation are two such forces. The ways in which they can interfere with the gratification of spiritual needs, and hence the attainment of an optimum state of health, well-being and quality of life, are illustrated in Figure 1.6.

It may be that the experience of illness/hospitalisation causes some individuals to face loss of control for the first time in their lives. As Granstrom (in Hitchens, 1988, p.26) states:

> Many individuals do not seriously search for the meaning and purpose of life but live as if life will go on for ever...Often it is not until the crisis, illness...or suffering occurs that the illusion (of security) is shattered...Therefore, illness, suffering...and ultimately death, by their very nature become spiritual encounters as well as physical and emotional experiences.

For many patients, therefore, spiritual care will be a necessary part of their total care.

This section has centred on describing and defining the spiritual dimension. It has been suggested that spiritual well-being and the meeting of spiritual needs, both in health and illness, are necessary for the maintenance of life itself and the attainment of an optimum state of health, well-being and quality of life. The experiences of illness and hospitalisation have been presented as crises which can precipitate spiritual distress and threaten the attainment of these goals. Given this, it is necessary to consider whether or not spiritual care should be part of the nurse's role (Chapter 4). As a prelude to this, an historical account of the changing philosophies of health care is given in Chapter 3.

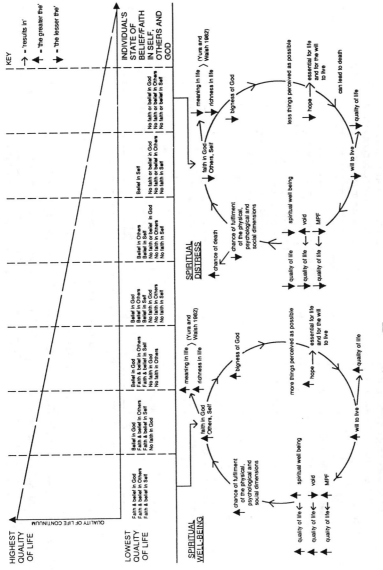

Figure 1.5 Quality of life continuum II

Source: Author's own

21

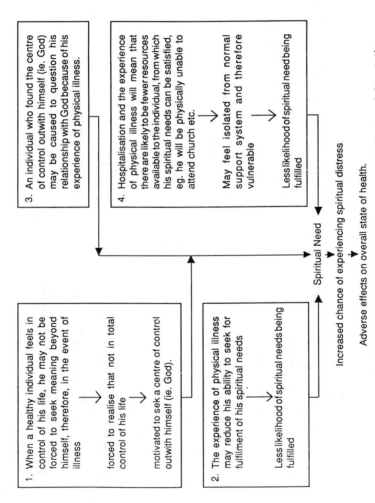

1. When a healthy individual feels in control of his life, he may not be forced to seek meaning beyond himself, therefore, in the event of illness

forced to realise that not in total control of his life

motivated to sek a centre of control outwith himself (ie. God).

2. The experience of physical illness may reduce his ability to seek for fulfilment of his spiritual needs

Less likelihood of spiritual needs being fulfilled

3. An individual who found the centre of control outwith himself (ie. God) may be caused to question his relationship with God because of his experience of physical illness.

4. Hospitalisation and the experience of physical illness will mean that there are likely to be fewer resources available to the individual, from which his spiritual needs can be satisfied, eg. he will be physically unable to attend church etc.

May feel isolated from normal support system and therefore vulnerable

Less likelihood of spiritual need being fulfilled

Spiritual Need

Increased chance of experiencing spiritual distress

Adverse effects on overall state of health.

Figure 1.6 Ways in which illness and hospitalisation can precipitate spiritual distress

Source: Author's own reprinted from the International Journal of Nursing Studies, 32, Ross, L. The spiritual dimension:its importance to patients health, well-being and quality of life and its implications for nursing practice, pp. 457-68, Copyright (1995), with kind permission from Elsevier Science Ltd, The Boulevard, Langford Lane, Kidlington, OX5 1GB, UK

Note

Sections of text on pp. 15, 17-19 author's own reproduced by kind permission of Blackwell Science Ltd from Ross (1994).

Sections of text on pp. 15, 17-19, 21 author's own reprinted from the International Journal of Nursing Studies, 32, Ross, L., The spiritual dimension: its importance to patients' health, well-being and quality of life and its implications for nursing practice, pp. 457-68, Copyright (1995), with kind permission from Elsevier Science Ltd, The Boulevard, Langford Lane, Kidlington OX5 1GB, UK.

3 Changing philosophies of health care: An historical overview

This chapter traces the changing philosophies of health care through the ages. It begins with the concept of humankind in its wholeness followed by the dualistic approach where physical and mental states were considered separately. Finally attention focuses on the slow re-emergence of the holistic concept today.

Most ancient civilisations were very much aware of the importance of phenomena, other than those directly observable, in influencing the disease process (Myco, 1985 a). Religion was one such acknowledged phenomenon, The individual's beliefs and relationship, or lack of them, with God, having a significant effect on health.

From as early as the fifth century B.C.,Hippocrates recognised that if the physician was truly to understand medicine, then he must also have a grasp of who and what humankind is. Thus, in traditional western medicine the body and soul were regarded as being inseparably linked, as evidenced by the way in which medical and spiritual care were provided within the one unit, e.g., 'Knights Hospitallers of St John' (Yura and Walsh, 1982). Plato (in Grubb 1977, p.33) stressed the danger of failing to provide total care when he stated:

this is the greatest error in the treatment of sickness, that there are physicians for the body and physicians for the soul - and yet the two are one and indivisible.

Even Nightingale herself (in Colliton, 1981, p.492), a pioneer in the emergence of nursing, in 1892, described nursing as a 'fine art' dealing with:

the living body - the temple of God's spirit.

However it was about a century ago that the importance attributed to the spiritual element was to change, the philosophy of care moving away from the holistic to the dualistic approach. It was here that the care of the spirit and physique gradually separated, the latter increasing in importance while the former declined, no longer assuming the significance it once had (Penrose and Barrett, 1982).

There are three main reasons for the divergence of care for the body and spirit, and the subsequent decline in importance of the latter. Each is discussed in turn below.

As a consequence of the rapid escalation in medical research, there emerged a period of enlightenment with regard to disease processes and treatments. As this approach relied heavily on measurable objective data, which the psychosocial and spiritual dimensions were incapable of producing, these dimensions of care gradually declined in importance. Meanwhile, medicine rapidly accumulated a wide range of knowledge from its proliferating research, which awed and captured the attention of the day, becoming virtually the sole concern with regard to health.

Secondly, pre-occupation with this approach has continued to spill over into modern medicine, which is increasingly gaining a powerful influence in areas of life from which it was previously banned. Zola (1978, p.254) has termed this process the 'medicalisation' of society, the implications of which are discussed below.

Although the importance accorded to medicine is hardly surprising, given that health scores so highly on society's list of values, it is also very disturbing as:

science is not the only path leading to the truth there being many others which will lead us further (Patey, 1963, p.3009).

The danger lies, not so much in the power and influence that medicine claims over health by its own contribution, but in the prevalence of the 'medical model', which views illness exclusively within the boundaries of physiological dysfunction (Ironbar, 1983). It is the fact that this approach excludes and denies the other dimensions of the individual and the contribution that they could make to the attainment of health, that is disturbing. As Nightingale (in Kramer, 1957, p.36) states:

the sick body...is something more than a reservoir for storing medicines.

Perhaps a greater danger than that of the medical model having assumed the right to define health and illness and determine what it considers to be the appropriate treatments, is that by considering only the individual's biological element, and even then differentiating it into smaller sub-units of study, the person is being treated as less than human by the mere fact that he/she is not being regarded in his/her wholeness (Moberg, 1979). Patient care consequently becomes fragmented and increasingly impersonal (Myco, 1985b).

Illich (1975) takes Zola's concept of the medicalisation of society further. He points out that the increasing variety of treatments provided by medicine, offering apparently unlimited improvement to health, can in fact have a negative effect. He has called this backlash of progress 'medical nemesis' or 'iatrogenesis'. An obvious example is the side effects of nausea, hair loss and lethargy caused by radiotherapy. However, iatrogenesis can be more insidious, e.g., the effects of institutionalisation. Perhaps Lewis (in Lecture Notes 101, p.2) had Illich's concept of nemesis in mind when he said:

man's power over nature is really the power of some men over other men, with nature as their instrument.

The third reason for the decline in the attention credited to the spiritual dimension, is the way in which the medical model has emphasised the process and mechanism of disease and illness, rather than the meaning of it (Fish and Shelly, 1978). As Nietsche (in Fish and Shelly, 1978, p.42) states, it is not the 'how' behind disease but the 'why' and the 'who' that is ultimately important. In other words, although it cannot be denied that the 'how' behind disease may be significant for its prevention and cure, what really matters is the meaning the individual can find in all life's experiences, including illness and death. According to Illich (1975) medicine has rendered illness, suffering and death meaningless. He cites this as another example of iatrogenesis.

It is clear that the approach of the scientific era, almost a century ago, and its development since then, resulted in a dualistic health care system, the consequence of which was that physiological care increased in importance while the spiritual dimension declined and even became an embarrassing subject. Although the medical model is still prevalent in health care today, the last 30 years have witnessed a rising recognition and concern that this approach to health is insufficient. This, together with the fear of the dehumanisation which could result from subdividing the individual into smaller and smaller fragments for the sake of scientific examination and discovery, has resulted in dissatisfaction with the medical model and consequently the re-emergence of the holistic concept (Hamel-Cooke and Cope, 1983).

Interest in the holistic concept of health is evidenced, first, by the emergence and rising popularity of complementary medicine (Peck, 1981). The recent shift in terminology from 'alternative' to 'complementary' medicine perhaps further emphasises the move toward holism. Techniques such as visualisation, biofeedback, massage and aromatherapy, to mention only a few examples, highlight the vital role played by the mind in controlling body processes (Burns, 1980, Rachman and Philips, 1978).

Secondly, there has been the introduction of the 'holistic' health care concept, where all aspects of the human being are regarded as important to his/her total state of well-being (Tubesing, 1979). Although this approach is more prominent in the USA, the central philosophy has been adopted in Britain's hospice movement, where spiritual care is given particular attention in the care of the dying.

The final example which highlights the desire to give holistic care, can be seen in the Marlebone project in London, where the clergy and medical staff collaborated in caring for the sick by forming a unit whose sole concern was to facilitate healing of the whole person (Hamel - Cooke and Cope, 1983).

In conclusion, from this historical account of the changing philosophies of health care, it is evident that the spiritual dimension has received varying degrees of attention over the years, depending on the particular conviction of society with regard to health at that time. Health care provision has thus come virtually full circle. It has moved from the rather mystical combination of religion and medicine in past centuries, to their divergence during the scientific era. Finally, their tendency to re-combine is evidenced by the way in which attention is swerving away from obsession with biological processes, in an effort to re-discover humankind in its wholeness.

4 Spiritual care: Should it be part of the nurse's role?

Having looked at how the concept of health care has changed over the years, the issue of whether or not spiritual care should be part of the nurse's role is addressed in this section. This is achieved by examining definitions of nursing, codes of conduct, models of nursing and guidelines for nurse education, each of which is discussed in turn.

Definitions of nursing

Definitions of nursing state that it is the responsibility of the nurse to:

promote health, to prevent illness, to restore health and to alleviate suffering (ICN, 1973).

assist the individual, sick or well, in the performance of those activities contributing to health or its recovery (or to a peaceful death) that he would perform unaided if he had the necessary strength, will or knowledge (Henderson, 1977, p.4).

Central to these definitions is the nurse's role in assisting patients to achieve their maximum health potential (Rogers, 1970 p.86). It has already been established that the level of health achieved by an individual will ultimately depend on the extent to which their spiritual needs are met. It is clear, therefore, that if nurses are to fulfil their function of promoting health, then spiritual care is a nursing responsibility and not an optional extra. It is necessary at this point to define spiritual care.

Nursing is a caring profession (Hargreaves, 1979) involving itself in helping patients meet needs conducive to health (Henderson, 1977). Given this, together with the fact that 'to take care of' has been defined as:

to make necessary arrangements regarding (Kirkpatrick, 1983, p.190)

spiritual care could be defined thus:

to make necessary arrangements for the provision of patients' spiritual needs.

In addition, a number of nursing authors such as Travelbee (1977) and Henderson (in Henderson and Nite, 1978) mention spiritual care explicitly. They acknowledge the need to find meaning in life and suffering which has already been identified as a spiritual need. Travelbee (in Fish and Shelly, 1979, p.59) goes further, however, and states that:

the existence of suffering whether physical mental or spiritual is the proper concern of the nurse.

Codes of conduct

Both national and international codes of conduct support spiritual care as a nursing responsibility.
Taking the former first, the UKCC states that it is the duty of the nurse to:

Take account of the customs, values and spiritual beliefs of patients/clients (UKCC, 1984 a, p.2).

Furthermore, it considers this to be:

a statement to the profession of the primacy of the interests of the patient or client (UKCC, 1984b, p.4) [which] places paramount importance upon the interests of patients and clients and the standard of their care (UKCC, 1991, p. 6) [and is] a portrait of the practitioner which the Council believes to be needed and which the Council wishes to see within the profession (UKCC, 1984b, p.4).

Thus the UKCC acknowledges that spiritual beliefs are of prime importance to the patient and that attention to these should similarly be reflected in nursing practice. A recent study conducted by the Nursing Times (Diamond, 1991) found that all Health Authorities, Health Boards and Trusts participating considered that the nurse had an obligation to work within the Code of Professional Conduct. The UKCC (1984b, p.4) also describes its pronouncement concerning nurses taking account of patients' spiritual beliefs, to be a:

clear unequivocal statement of the profession's values (UKCC 1984b, p.4).

However, rather than being 'clear', this declaration appears rather ambiguous. For instance 'to take account of' could be interpreted in a rather passive way where the nurse is not actively involved in helping patients meet their spiritual needs. Alternatively, it could be interpreted to mean the nurse being actively involved in helping patients with these needs. Furthermore, the definition of 'spiritual beliefs' is open to interpretation. For example, it could be viewed in terms of religious beliefs only or in the broader context including the needs for MPF, hope, etc.

Concerning international codes of conduct, the ICN (1973), considers its Code for Nurses to be:

a guide for action based on values and needs of society.

and states that

The nurse, in providing care, promotes an environment in which the values, customs and spiritual beliefs of the individual are respected.

Thus the spiritual beliefs of the individual are recognised and valued by the Council, so much so that this is reflected in its guidelines for nursing practice. However it is unclear what is actually meant by 'respecting' patients' 'spiritual beliefs' and 'promoting an environment' in which this can be achieved. The ICN (1977, p.14) considers the nurse:

best able to assess the operating...beliefs and incorporate her knowledge of them in directing the nursing care.

This suggests an active rather than a passive role for the nurse in respecting patients' spiritual beliefs. Perhaps this lack of clarity is due to the fact that the Code does not purport to act as a law but rather as a guide providing nurses with:

a broad statement of the nurse's responsibility as a professional person (ICN 1977, p.vii).

Because it was unclear what the UKCC and ICN meant by their statements, the researcher wrote to them to ask for an explanation. Neither organisation could give this, however, it is worthy of note that the statements concerning patients' spiritual beliefs had been added to the Codes. The UKCC's statement was considered a necessary addition because the Council felt that practitioners often ignore patients' spiritual needs. Concerning the ICN, their statement was added to the Code following its review in 1973.

It would appear, therefore, that codes of conduct acknowledge spiritual care as a necessary and valued part of the nurse's role. Although it is not clear what is actually expected of the nurse, the fact that in both cases these were additions to the Codes perhaps reflects increasing recognition of the influence of the spiritual dimension on health and illness as suggested in Chapter 3.

Models of nursing

Models of nursing include consideration of the spiritual dimension either directly or by ascribing to the individual's wholeness and search for meaning.

Considering those which do so directly, Henderson states that it is the duty of the nurse to assist the patient to:

worship according to his faith (Henderson, 1977, p.13).

and:

practice his religion or conform to his concept of right and wrong (Henderson, 1977, p.19).

She interprets spiritual need in the religious context and contends that if religious practice is essential to the individual's sense of well-being in health, then it will be all the more necessary during illness.

Ways in which she suggests the nurse can help patients practise their religion are by:

1 Enabling them to attend a place of worship.
2 Contacting and involving appropriate clergy in the patient's care.
3 Providing privacy for patient and clergy.
4 Making necessary arrangements for them to receive the sacraments.

Watson (in Riehl-Sisca, 1989) also includes the spiritual dimension in her model of nursing. Rather than concentrating on the religious aspect she views spirituality in the broader context of the individual's need for meaning and harmony in existence and for transcendence to a higher level of consciousness. She postulates that if the individual is to experience true wholeness, then he/she must live in contact with and feed their soul/spirit which is the very core of their being. It is through the soul that the individual can transcend the here and now and co-exist simultaneously with the past, present and future, thereby becoming fully integrated and self-actualised. These are similar ideas to those of Brewer (1979) and Maslow (in DiCaprio, 1974) presented in Chapter 2. According to Watson, disease/illness can cause or be caused by disharmony in the individual's inner self. The goal of nursing is, therefore, to assist them to achieve inner harmony from which will emanate self healing. This can be achieved through the 'caring' action of the nurse who is required to be sensitive in order to nurture faith and hope in the patient.

Both Rogers (in Riehl-Sisca, 1989) and Weidenbach (in Fitzpatrick and Whall, 1983) give consideration to the spiritual dimension by ascribing to the individual's wholeness, of which the spiritual is part.

Fitzpatrick's Rhythm Model (in Fitzpatrick and Whall, 1983) includes consideration of the spiritual dimension by concentrating on search for meaning which has already been identified as a spiritual need.

Other models such as Roy's Adaptation Model and Neuman's Health Care Systems Model, have been criticised (in Riehl-Sisca, 1989) for failing to incorporate the spiritual dimension overtly. Some authors have, therefore, adapted them to include this.

Guidelines for nurse education

Finally, both British and international guidelines for nurse education indicate that spiritual care should be taught to nurses.

Taking the UK first, in preparation for Project 2000 it has been recommended that nurse education should:

> provide opportunities to enable the student to...acquire the competencies required to: xiv) identify...spiritual needs of the patient or client, devise a plan of care, contribute to its implementation and evaluation by demonstrating an appreciation and practice of principles of a problem solving approach. (UKCC, 1986, pp. 40-41).

This is further reflected in Scotland in the NBS's consideration of the reforms for basic nurse education. Amongst its aims and objectives is that the nurse will be enabled to:

> assess, plan, implement and evaluate care to meet the...spiritual...needs of the individual and family/ friends. (NBS, 1990, p.16).

In short, in the UK, nursing students are to be taught how to give spiritual care using the nursing process.

On the international scene the ICN (1973) which, as stated previously, includes spiritual care in its Code for Nurses, considers the Code:

> will have meaning only if it becomes a living document applied to the realities of human behaviour in a changing society... In order to achieve its purpose the Code must be put before and be continuously available to students...throughout their study and work lives.

Furthermore the AACN (1986, p.5) recommends that the education of the professional nurse should ensure his/her ability to:

> Comprehend the meaning of human spirituality in order to recognise the relationship of beliefs to culture, behaviour, health and healing.

and to plan and implement this care.

In conclusion, having examined definitions of nursing, codes of conduct, models of nursing and guidelines for nurse education, it is suggested that spiritual care is a nursing responsibility and not an optional extra. This raises the question of whether or not nurses actually practise spiritual care. This issue is addressed in Chapter 5.

5   Spiritual care: Is it practised by nurses?

Having illustrated that spiritual care should be part of the nurse's role, attention now focuses on whether or not this would appear to be the case in practice. This is achieved by reviewing the current nursing literature and research with regard to spiritual care.

A review of the literature

Five books were located which are specifically devoted to spiritual care in nursing. Three are American. Two of these are written by nurses affiliated with the Nurses Christian Fellowship (NCF) (Fish and Shelly, 1978, Shelly and John, 1983). The majority of contributors in the other publication are nurse educators based predominantly in the nursing department of one university (Carson, 1989).

The two other books are British. The most recent is written by a nurse tutor (Narayanasamy, 1991) and the other contributed to mainly by nurse educators in Northern Ireland but also clergy (McGilloway and Myco, 1985).

Concerning the content of the books, those of Fish and Shelly (1978) and Shelly and John (1983) are written predominantly from a Christian perspective. Although they are somewhat vague, they provided the launch pad for future literature on the subject. Those of McGilloway and Myco (1985) and Carson (1989) are the most comprehensive giving an historical account of spirituality, outlining the religious practices relevant to different faiths and applying spiritual care to different settings e.g., acute illness, giving specific patient examples. Furthermore, in Carson's (1989) book there is a good overview of the concepts of spirituality, spiritual need, spiritual well-being and spiritual distress.

Some other nursing texts were found to contain chapters on spirituality. A British text by Henderson and Nite (1978) contains a chapter entitled 'Worship' which concentrates mainly on religious aspects of spirituality. Other American texts such as Murray and Zentner (1975) and Beland and Passos (1975) include chapters which basically summarise the information presented in the books specifically on spiritual care.

In addition to text books, there has been a proliferation in the number of journal articles written on spiritual care in recent years, as can be seen from the reference list. Most of these articles are anecdotal. Few are research based and most are American.

In summary, having reviewed the literature on spiritual care, it would appear that the majority of texts agree that nurses should be giving spiritual care, however, operational definitions of 'spiritual' and 'spiritual need' are lacking as are guidelines for the practice of spiritual care.

A review of nursing research on spiritual care

It would appear that research is very much in its infancy, few studies having been undertaken. Furthermore, the ability to generalise findings is limited by the fact that the majority of studies are American in origin. Only two British studies were identified (Chomicz, 1984; Simsen, 1985) neither of which looked at the nurse's perspective. Also, in addition to the fact that many of these studies are now rather outdated, most researchers used small samples of convenience and tools which had not been tested for reliability or validity. Moreover comparison between studies is made difficult by the fact that operational definitions of terms are frequently lacking or are not cited in summarised versions of the original studies. There is no guarantee, therefore, that the terminology used is consistent across studies.

Bearing these limitations in mind, an overview is given below of this small, but growing, body of research by looking first at studies which address the patient's perspective of spiritual need and spiritual care followed by those concerned with nurses' opinions and nurse education.

Five studies were identified which looked at the patient's perspective on spiritual need and spiritual care. These are presented in chronological order.

Study 1

In 1969 Stallwood-Hess endeavoured to determine patients' awareness of their spiritual needs. Twelve nurses from the NCF interviewed 109 patients who were not critically ill. These patients were selected from a number of hospitals and had been in-patients for three or more days. Examples of questions asked were:

1 Were you aware of having a spiritual need at any time during your hospitalisation?

2 Has your need been met to any degree or is it still present?

The findings revealed that spiritual needs expressed by patients were for, in rank order:

1 Prayer.
2 Relief from loneliness.
3 Awareness of God's presence.
4 Relief from fear of surgery and death.
5 Meaning and purpose in life, death and suffering.
6 Relief from guilt, loss of faith, doubt.
7 Expression of their faith by visible means.

It was not reported whether or not any patients had stated that they experienced no spiritual needs.

Patients sought assistance with meeting their needs first from the clergy followed by the nurse, then others such as family and friends. The majority were satisfied with the help they had received. Others indicated that their need had only been partially met whilst some (10%) had received no help at all.

When asked how they thought nurses could help them with their spiritual needs, some felt nurses were too busy whilst others stated they could help by:

1 Listening.
2 Referring to the chaplain.
3 Talking with them.
4 Praying with them.
5 'Being there'.

Thus, although Stallwood-Hess's study was limited by the fact that several interviewers were used, all of whom belonged to the NCF which could have introduced interviewer bias, it would appear that, within the sample, patients experienced spiritual needs while in hospital. These needs were, however, not always entirely met. Furthermore, patients considered the nurse to have a significant role in spiritual care.

Study 2

Kealey (1974) interviewed 40 patients randomly selected from medical and surgical wards in four hospitals in a mid-western city in the USA, to determine what they perceived their spiritual needs to be. Interviews lasted between 30-60 minutes and included 45 questions.

She found that the majority of patients (60%) reported no spiritual needs during hospitalisation. Of those who did, needs they experienced included:

1 Relief from fear of surgery, pain, dying.
2 Relief from loneliness.
3 Support from clergy.
4 Help to accept poor prognosis.
5 Reassurance of having made the right decision.
6 Someone to listen and understand.
7 Opportunity to participate in worship services.

Some patients would have liked spiritual help from the nurse, however, the majority did not see this as part of the nurse's duty. No patients had received help with their spiritual needs from the nurse but rather met their needs alone or with help from family, friends or clergy.

Kealey concluded that it should not be assumed that just because a person is hospitalised they will have spiritual needs. She acknowledged, however, that for some patients, having their spiritual needs attended to will be important.

Study 3

Martin et al. (1976) also sought to determine the spiritual needs hospitalised patients experienced. They used a self completion questionnaire combined with an interview to retrieve this information from 65 adults in two area general hospitals in the USA. Just under half (48%) of these patients said they had experienced spiritual needs such as for:

1 Support.
2 Hope.
3 Relief from fear.
4 Comfort.
5 Meaning in suffering.
6 Relationship with God.

They had discussed their needs in the first instance with the clergy, then with family followed by the nurse. Whilst 29% felt their need had not been met, the majority considered it had been met in part.

Patients considered that nurses could give spiritual care by:

1 Listening.
2 Referring to the clergy.
3 Showing kindness, understanding.
4 'Being there'.

However the majority of patients felt that nurses did not have enough time to do so.

Study 4

Chomicz (1984) sought to investigate patients' experiences of spiritual need by conducting semi-structured interviews with a volunteer sample of 30 orthopaedic patients from three wards in a London teaching hospital.

She found that 29 out of 30 patients stated they had experienced a spiritual need during their hospitalisation. The most commonly cited needs were (in rank order):

1 For help to trust God more.
2 Lack of peace.
3 Lack of meaning in suffering.
4 Loneliness.

Half would have been glad to talk to a nurse about their need and the majority had not seen a chaplain but would have liked to.

Study 5

Simsen (1985) conducted 45 semi-structured interviews with patients in general medical and surgical wards in England. She found that illness and hospitalisation posed a threat to their physical integrity, confidence and personal relatedness. Religious practices e.g., prayer, were highly valued by many patients and helped them to find meaning in their experience.

In summary, from the patient's viewpoint, with the exception of one study (Kealey 1974), nursing research indicates that for many patients illness and hospitalisation can become spiritual encounters as suggested in Figure 1.6. During these experiences a considerable proportion of patients reported spiritual needs (Chomicz, 1984, Martin et al., 1976, Stallwood-Hess, 1969) and furthermore considered these of importance to them (Simsen, 1985).

Some patients would have liked nurses to help them with their spiritual needs by such actions as listening, 'being there' and referring to the clergy where appropriate (Chomicz, 1984, Kealey, 1974, Martin et al., 1976, Stallwood-Hess, 1969) however, many felt that the nurse was too busy to help in these ways.

Commonly expressed were the needs for: meaning; belief in God, often expressed through formal religious practices; relief from fear, doubt, loneliness; relatedness to others/God.

Although patients tended to express satisfaction with the assistance they had received (in Martin et al.'s, 1976 study the majority were completely satisfied) Stallwood-Hess (1969) found that the majority felt their needs had not been met to the full. Furthermore, chaplains reported that, despite receiving excellent physical care, patients were often found to be struggling to grasp the meaning of their suffering (Bowlby, 1980, Patey, 1977).

Given that hospitalised patients considered their spiritual needs of importance, it would seem appropriate, therefore, that nurses should endeavour to help patients meet these needs. An overview of the research related to the nurse's perspective of spiritual care is given below.

Six American studies, dating from as early as 1957, sought to obtain nurses' opinions of spiritual care and their role in this.

Study 1

In 1957 Kramer distributed questionnaires to 83 practising registered nurses in Oregon obtaining a 94% response rate. Details of the sampling method are somewhat sparse and the information sought was exclusively related to nurses' knowledge of various religious practices.

She found that, although the majority of nurses considered spiritual care part of total nursing care (93.6%), only 56.4% felt able to give this in practice. Nurses generally had a limited understanding of religious practices. Those who indicated the greatest ability to provide spiritual care had been in practice in excess of ten years.

Study 2

Chance (1967) administered a questionnaire to 37 senior student nurses asking them about their identification of patients' spiritual needs. As all students were from Seventh Day Adventist Colleges, the results may be somewhat biased.

The majority of students (73%) said they had identified spiritual needs which included the need for faith and hope in and for love of God. They recognised these needs mainly through non-verbal cues given by patients and responded by listening, praying with/reading the Bible to the patient or by contacting the chaplain.

Study 3

In 1973 Chadwick distributed questionnaires to a random sample of nurses working in the Michigan area. The sample size is not stated, however the results are based on 34 returns. Again the emphasis was on religious needs.

All nurses felt that patients had spiritual needs and all stated they had identified at least one need.

Although half said they had never read the Bible to a patient, the majority of nurses (75%) said they would feel comfortable doing so. Over half (57.6%) felt patients' spiritual needs were adequately met, whereas 33.3% felt they were poorly met.

Furthermore, although the majority (81.8%) felt they had some knowledge of religious practices, most (60.6%) expressed the desire for further education in this respect.

Study 4

The second part of Kealey's (1974) study examined the nurse's perception of her role in spiritual care. Of the 24 questionnaires distributed to registered nurses, seventeen were returned. The responses revealed that, although the majority (91%) of nurses considered it was part of their duty to assist patients of various faiths to meet their spiritual needs, just over half felt able to do so. Appropriate activities reported by them were listening, reading religious literature if asked and referring to the clergy.

Study 5

Highfield and Cason (1983) distributed a questionnaire to 100 surgical nurses working in a large south western private hospital in order to examine their awareness of patients' spiritual needs. Based on the low response rate of 35%, they found that these nurses had a limited awareness of patients' spiritual needs. Only those behaviours related to specific religious beliefs and practices were identified with the spiritual dimension and these were thought to occur infrequently. (Similarly Fish and Shelly (1978) noted how, in practice, nurses placed primary importance on physical care, secondary importance on the psychosocial realm, but rarely considered the spiritual dimension.)

Although just over half (53%) had received education on spiritual care in their basic training (the nature or extent of this was not clear), few felt their greatest need was for further education in this area. Almost all expressed the desire for more teaching on psychosocial care.

Study 6

In a study of 300 registered nurses practising throughout the USA, Piles (1986) found that 96.5% considered holistic care to include spiritual care. Whilst 87.6% disagreed that only clergy could give spiritual care, 65.9% felt inadequately prepared to provide this. The nursing diagnosis of spiritual distress was used by 13% and 11% included spiritual needs, goals and interventions in nursing care plans. Few had been taught about spiritual care in their basic education programme, 78% felt that if they had known then they would have been able to give spiritual care and 89.2% agreed that spiritual care should be included in basic nurse education.

Factors found to be significant (at .001 level) in determining whether or not nurses gave spiritual care were:

1 The nurse's perceived ability to provide care.
2 The degree of educational input in the nurse's basic programme.
3 The degree of importance the nurse placed on spiritual care.
4 Obstacles the nurse perceived in providing spiritual care, e.g., lack of time.

In conclusion, research indicates that nurses were aware patients had spiritual needs (100% and 96.5% in the studies of Chadwick, 1973 and Piles, 1986 respectively) the majority (93.6%, 91% and 75% in Kramer, 1957, Kealey, 1974 and Chadwick, 1973 respectively) regarding it their duty to make provision for at least some of these needs. Furthermore, according to Piles (1986) 87.6% of nurses disagreed that spiritual care was the remit of the clergy only. Despite this, however, it would appear that nurses had a limited ability to attend to the spiritual needs of patients.

Although Chance (1967) found that the majority of student nurses identified spiritual needs, these results may be somewhat biased. In addition, the basis on which over half the nurses in Chadwick's (1973) study concluded that patients' spiritual needs had been adequately met was unclear.

It is the general consensus of other studies, however, that despite the fact that nurses usually displayed some knowledge of and ability to identify the more obvious, direct religious needs e.g., for communion (Chadwick, 1973) they were less aware of spiritual needs than those pertaining to the psychosocial dimension (Highfield and Cason, 1983). Moreover they demonstrated a limited knowledge of and ability to help patients meet their spiritual needs (Highfield and Cason, 1983, Kramer, 1957).

Furthermore, Kramer (1957), Kealey (1974) and Piles (1986) found that whilst 93.6%, 91% and 87.6% of nurses agreed that spiritual care was a nursing responsibility, only 56.4%, 50% and 34.1% respectively felt able to provide for this adequately. This was a similar finding to Chadwick (1973) who also noted that, despite the fact that 75% of nurses stated that they would feel comfortable reading the Bible to or praying with patients, only 50% actually did so in practice. Additionally, in Kealey's (1974) study, patients with spiritual needs received no help from nurses.

The inadequacy felt by nurses in providing spiritual care was further borne out by the fact that, with the exception of Highfield and Cason's (1983) study, many expressed the need for further education in the meeting of such needs (Chadwick, 1973, Piles, 1986).

Therefore, generally, it would appear that practising nurses, cited in the aforementioned studies, expressed the desire to be involved in giving spiritual care but felt inadequate in providing this.

With regard to spiritual care in nurse education it appeared that the teaching of spiritual care to nurses was a necessary pre-requisite to its practice by them. No research, however, could be identified which tested this assumption.

Furthermore, it seemed to be generally assumed that spiritual care was not taught, however, few research studies, certainly no British ones, were identified which addressed this issue. The author, therefore, enquired of all basic nurse education establishments in Scotland with regard to their teaching input on spiritual care. This took the form of a letter of enquiry to the person in charge of the establishment. From the responses received it would appear that spiritual care does not form a substantial identifiable component in any education programme e.g., it may take the form of a one hour session from the hospital chaplain and be touched upon in religious practices in care of the dying.

Moves are being made, however, in the area of curriculum development. Piles (1986) postulated that three aspects must be present for learning to occur: student; setting; subject of study. She contended, however, that although the student may be present, the ward setting often discourages the practice of spiritual care and the teaching of spiritual care is often absent from nurse education programmes.

As early as 1957 Lewis set about developing a resource unit for the inclusion of spiritual care in the basic nursing curriculum at the University of Washington School of Nursing. Twenty volunteer students worked on a variety of spiritual care studies. Later, Hitchens (1988) found that students tended to project themes from their own faith, values and life experiences into patient care situations. Furthermore, rather than length of experience, life experience/crisis was a major factor in determining the level of the student's faith development (as measured by an interview developed by Fowler) which in turn appeared to influence the way in which students planned spiritual care. In addition, interpersonal skills e.g., therapeutic use of self, were considered important by these students in giving spiritual care.

In conclusion the lack of research and literature on the teaching of spiritual care in nurse education programmes, together with the findings from a brief survey conducted in Scotland, tend to indicate that it is a subject not taught to any degree in basic nurse education programmes. This contradicts the recommendations, outlined in Chapter 4, given for nurse education.

To summarise this section it would appear there is a lack of literature on spiritual care. The available literature is largely anecdotal, fails to reach a generally agreed definition of what is meant by 'spiritual', 'spiritual need' and 'spiritual care' and omits to give nurses guidelines for practice. There is a distinct lack of research on spiritual care, particularly of British origin. Bearing in mind the limitations of available studies, it would appear that patients experience spiritual needs but often these needs are not fully met, the implications of which could be serious as illustrated in Figure 1.7. In addition, patients consider that the nurse could have a significant role in giving spiritual care and nurses appear to be willing to do so but feel inadequate in this regard. Also, it would seem that, despite the fact that guidelines for education advocate the teaching of spiritual care, this does not occur to any great extent.

Note

Sections of text on pp. 40-41 author's own reprinted from the International Journal of Nursing Studies, 32, Ross, L., The spiritual dimension: its importance to patients' health, well-being and quality of life and its implications for nursing practice, p.p. 457-68, Copyright (1995), with kind permission from Elsevier Science Ltd, The Boulevard, Langford Lane, Kidlington OX5 1GB, UK.

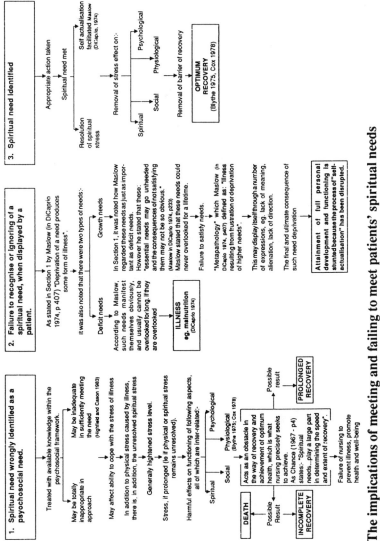

Figure 1.7 The implications of meeting and failing to meet patients' spiritual needs

Source: Author's own reprinted from the International Journal of Nursing Studies, 32, Ross, L. The spiritual dimension:its importance to patients health, well-being and quality of life and its implications for nursing practice, pp. 457-68, Copyright (1995), with kind permission from Elsevier Science Ltd, The Boulevard, Langford Lane, Kidlington, OX5 1GB, UK

6 Summary

In summary, having illustrated the influence of the spiritual dimension on health, well-being and quality of life (Chapter 2) and having established that spiritual care is a nursing responsibility (Chapters 3 and 4), evidence has been presented which tends to indicate that patients' spiritual needs may not be well attended to in practice (Chapter 5). Although moves have been made to contribute to the knowledge base for spiritual care, this is very much in its infancy and nurses currently lack guidelines for practice.

Part Two
PROPOSED CONCEPTUAL FRAMEWORK FOR GIVING SPIRITUAL CARE EMERGING FROM THE LITERATURE

7 Proposed conceptual framework

Part 1 illustrated how there appeared to be insufficient knowledge and guidelines to enable nurses to give spiritual care. This Part proposes a conceptual framework for giving spiritual care based on the nursing process (Figure 2.1) and is explained below.

An individual entering hospital will do so with a particular spiritual orientation. As described in Part 1, the experience of illness/hospitalisation may cause them to experience spiritual needs for the first time in their life or to experience new dimensions of spiritual need. Alternatively, spiritual needs which were a part of the individual's life prior to admission will continue throughout their hospitalisation. It is likely, therefore, that many people will experience spiritual needs when they become patients. Whether or not these needs are met may determine the speed and extent of their recovery and the level of spiritual well-being and quality of life they experience while in hospital. It is important, therefore, that they receive the necessary help to meet their spiritual needs.

One way of ensuring that patients' spiritual needs are met is by using the nursing process as the mechanism to deliver systematic individualised spiritual care (Kratz, 1979, Marriner, 1988). This will involve identifying the patient's spiritual needs through conducting a spiritual assessment, planning and implementing the appropriate interventions to meet these needs and evaluating to what extent these interventions have been successful. At the outset this seems fairly simple. However, on closer examination it would appear that in order for each stage of the nursing process to be enacted, it will be necessary to have the following knowledge:

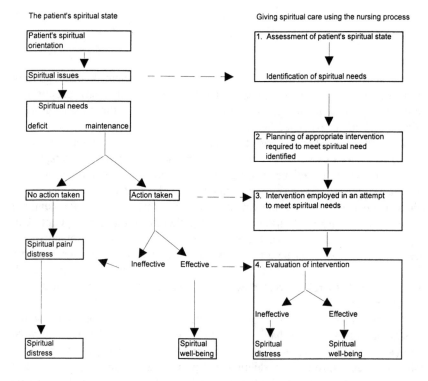

The patient's spiritual state

Patient's spiritual orientation

Spiritual issues

Spiritual needs

deficit   maintenance

No action taken   Action taken

Spiritual pain/ distress

Ineffective   Effective

Spiritual distress

Spiritual well-being

Giving spiritual care using the nursing process

1. Assessment of patient's spiritual state

Identification of spiritual needs

2. Planning of appropriate intervention required to meet spiritual need identified

3. Intervention employed in an attempt to meet spiritual needs

4. Evaluation of intervention

Ineffective   Effective

Spiritual distress

Spiritual well-being

Figure 2.1 A proposed conceptual framework for giving spiritual care using the nursing process

Source: Author's own reproduced by kind permission of Blackwell
             Science Ltd. from Ross (1994)

Stage of Nursing Process	Knowledge required
Assessment	What spiritual needs are. How they can be recognised, i..e., indicators of spiritual distress.
Planning Intervention	What might be appropriate interventions for the meeting of these needs.
Evaluation	What factors would indicate that the needs had been met, i.e., spiritual well-being indicators.

To ensure continuity, it would be important to document spiritual care in the patient's care plan. Each stage of the nursing process applied to spiritual care is addressed in turn.

Assessment

Part 1 highlighted the absence of a generally agreed definition of 'spiritual' or 'spiritual need'. This makes it difficult to conduct an assessment. In recent years, however, moves have been made toward developing spiritual assessment tools.

Stoll (1979), in her 'Guidelines for Spiritual Assessment' identified four areas for assessment. These included the patient's: concept of God/deity; source of hope and strength; religious practices and rituals; perception of relationship between spiritual beliefs and state of health.

Questions she suggested as useful in exploring the above include:

1 Is religion or God significant for you?
2 To whom do you turn when you need help?
3 Do you feel your faith (religion) is helpful to you? If yes tell me how?
4 Has being sick (or what happened to you) made any difference in your feeling about God or the practise of your faith?

She advocates that the spiritual assessment be placed at the end of the general assessment.

Also, in 1973 Fish and Williams (in Hitchens, 1988) developed tools with similar questions and in 1984 Still devised a version for use with children (in Hitchens, 1988).

In addition to the development of spiritual assessment tools by nurses, another major area of expansion has been the introduction of the concept of nursing diagnosis. The notion was developed from Henderson's fourteen basic needs and is defined by Carpenito (in Hitchens, 1988, p.29) as:

> a statement that describes a health state or an actual or potential alteration in one's life processes (physiological, psychological, socio-cultural, developmental and spiritual).

Since its inception in 1973, NANDA has developed more than 60 diagnostic categories, one of which is spiritual distress (distress of the human spirit) (Kim et al., 1984, p.57). This has been defined as:

> a disruption in the life principle that pervades a person's entire being and that integrates and transcends one's biologic and psychosocial nature.

The diagnosis can be made in relation to the individual's need for forgiveness, love, hope, trust, meaning and purpose and for each need a list of indicators is given.

Spiritual distress indicators were also used by Highfield and Cason (1983) in relation to the needs: for meaning and purpose; to give and receive love; for hope and creativity and were developed from Clinebell's 'religious-existential' framework. The concept of spiritual distress is termed 'spiritual problems' by Highfield and Cason (1983).

It would appear, therefore, that some developments have been made in the realm of assessing patients' spiritual needs, although as far as the researcher is aware, measures have not yet been employed to test these for validity and reliability.

Planning and intervention

Whereas few would argue against nurses assessing patients' spiritual needs and evaluating the care given, disparity appears to exist with regard to whether or not all nurses should be actively involved in responding to patients' spiritual needs.

It is the opinion of most authors that nurses should respond to patients' spiritual needs (Fish and Shelly, 1978, Piles, 1986). However, De Young (in Hitchens, 1988, p.43) is doubtful about this and perhaps reflects the opinions of other nurses in her statement:

> I am not convinced the nursing profession should assume the role of meeting patients' spiritual needs. Christian nurses...and perhaps other

nurses interested in spiritual matters do have a role in spiritual care. But the fact that some nurses choose to provide spiritual care does not mean that all nurses should.

De Young, however, agrees that all nurses should assess spiritual needs but may refer them elsewhere to be met. As shown in Part 1 there are few guidelines to indicate what might be appropriate and inappropriate interventions for meeting patients' spiritual needs.

Evaluation

Little is known about factors which would indicate that a patient's spiritual needs had been met. Highfield and Cason (1983) used some indicators based on Clinebell's work, but again it is not clear if these were tested for validity and reliability.

Studies conducted both in the UK (O'Neill, 1984) and the USA (Hitchens, 1988) tend to indicate that spiritual care is not documented in patients' care plans.

In summary, it would appear that there is a lack of knowledge with regard to what spiritual needs are, how spiritual care may be given and how it can be evaluated which makes it difficult for nurses to give it using the framework of the nursing process. Further research is clearly required to contribute to the knowledge base which would enable spiritual care to be given in this way. However, even if this knowledge was available, nurses may still be reluctant to give spiritual care as indicated by De Young's statement above. There is evidence to suggest that a variety of factors may determine the nurse's ability/willingness to give spiritual care. These include:

1   The way in which the nurse defines the spiritual dimension (Highfield and Cason, 1983) and the importance she places on spiritual care (Hitchens, 1988, Piles, 1986).

2   The nurse's perception of: whose responsibility spiritual care is (Hitchens, 1988); her ability to meet patients' spiritual needs (Piles, 1986); the obstacles preventing her from responding (Piles, 1986).

3   The teaching the nurse has received on spiritual care (Hitchens, 1988; Piles, 1986).

Over-riding all these factors, however, would appear to be the value system of the nurse in determining her ability to give spiritual care. Several authors and researchers cite the degree to which the nurse is aware of, is secure in and has developed her own spiritual quest, as central to her ability to function in giving spiritual care. Many authors have suggested that the nurse's life experience, particularly in the form of crisis, may act as a force for spiritual growth (Granstrom, 1985, Hitchens, 1988, Kreidler, 1984 in Hitchens, 1988, Shelly and John, 1978, Vaillot, 1970).

Thus, most of the above authors and others advocate the teaching of spiritual self awareness to nursing students as a means of educating them on spiritual care. All of these authors were American. No comparable British work was identified. However, in her study of a sample of district nurses in Britain, Hockey (1979) discovered that the care these nurses gave was not entirely dictated by patients' needs but by a variety of other factors, such as personal characteristics of the nurse, her social background and professional preparation as well as work-related factors such as administrative concerns and the influence of other professionals (Figure 2.2). Although not directly related to spiritual care, the finding is similar to that cited by previous American authors where personal characteristics of the nurse and her professional preparation influenced the care she gave.

In summary, it was noted that guidelines to enable nurses to give spiritual care were lacking. This chapter has suggested a conceptual framework for the giving of spiritual care using the nursing process. It is acknowledged, however, that further research is required to produce the necessary knowledge for this framework to become operational and even then, that the ability/willingness of the nurse to give spiritual care might be determined by other factors.

Note

Sections of text on p.p. 15, 17-19 author's own reproduced by kind permission of Blackwell Science Ltd from Ross (1994).

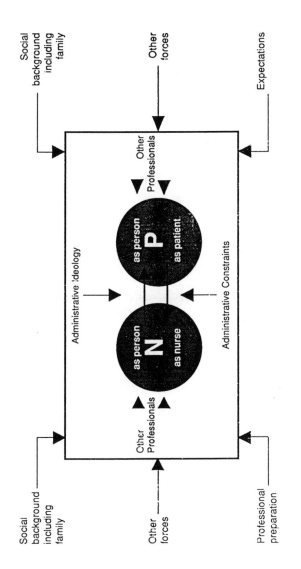

Figure 2.2 Conceptual model of factors influencing nursing care
Source: Hockey (1979). Reproduced by kind permission of Dr Hockey

Part Three
OVERVIEW OF THE STUDY

8 Purpose

This brief chapter outlines the purpose of the study, details how the population was selected and gives an overview of the general approach adopted for conducting the study.

Having reviewed the literature, it is evident that spiritual care is part of the nurse's role (Part 1). Little British research on spiritual care and few guidelines for its practice were, however, identified (Part 2). Given the importance of spiritual well-being to the attainment of an optimum state of health, together with the fact that the extent to which a patient achieves this will be determined by the nursing care given, it was considered important to gain some insight into how nurses perceive spiritual care and their role in this. Furthermore, the literature review highlighted that a variety of factors may influence how nurses give spiritual care (Parts 1 and 2). This exploratory, descriptive study sought, therefore, to address the following research questions:

1 How do nurses perceive spiritual need and spiritual care and report to give the latter in practice?

2 What factors appear to influence the spiritual care given to patients?

9 Selection of the population

The population of nurses intended for inclusion in the study consisted of staff nurses (S/N's) and charge nurses (C/N's) working full-time day or night duty on non-psychiatric care of the elderly wards situated within general and geriatric NHS hospitals in Scotland. The rationale for each criterion is given below.

S/N's and C/N's

To minimise the effects that differing levels of qualification could have had on the results (as would have been the case had enrolled or student nurses been included), only those nurses who had achieved a first level qualification in nursing (RGN or SRN) were included.

Working full-time day or night duty

As nothing was known about the prevalence of spiritual needs only full-time staff were included in an attempt to ensure that all nurses had equal opportunity to identify these needs. In addition, as it was thought that spiritual needs may be more evident at night, both day and night staff were included.

Employed on non-psychiatric care of the elderly wards

Care of the elderly settings were chosen as it was thought that spiritual needs may be easier to identify if nurses had had opportunity to get to know their patients. Psychogeriatric wards were excluded as it was suspected that the condition of such patients might make the identification of spiritual needs difficult.

Working in general and geriatric NHS hospitals

The above hospitals were selected to minimise the possible influence that special resources/training (e.g., hospice care specifically designed to meet the needs of the dying or special facilities provided by private hospitals/homes) might have had on the findings. In order to ascertain if there was any difference in the spiritual care given in general and geriatric hospitals, both were included for comparison.

Hospitals situated in Scotland

Scotland was chosen for the following reasons:

1   It provided an already existing natural division within the UK.

2   A manageable size of population could be obtained by including all Health Boards, any geographical differences found in nurses' perceptions/ giving of spiritual care could be detected.

3 Any differences in culture, nursing administration and nurse training between Scotland and England (Scotland having its own National Board), which may have affected results and made the procedure for gaining access more complicated, could be minimised.

10 Approach adopted for the study

In order to address the research questions, a blend of both quantitative and qualitative approaches was adopted. Chalmers (1989, p.37) states:

> because the strengths of one methodology are often the weaknesses of the other, research that seeks to draw on the strengths of each may maximise the reliability and validity of the results.

It was considered that by using more than one method to collect and interpret data a more accurate representation of how spiritual care was actually perceived and practised by nurses and the factors influencing this care would be obtained. Thus the study was undertaken in two separate but related parts.

In part one (quantitative) a purpose designed postal questionnaire was selected as the method which would elicit basic information from a large number of nurses distributed over a wide geographical area in relation to their perceptions and giving of spiritual care. In part two (qualitative), it was considered that a semi-structured interview would allow for deeper exploration of nurses' perceptions and practice of spiritual care and would create the opportunity for further investigation of factors thought to influence how spiritual care was given. Parts 4 and 5 describe the quantitative and qualitative approaches respectively.

Part Four
QUANTITATIVE APPROACH

11 Aims

Part 4 describes the quantitative approach. First, the research questions are outlined and the method selected for addressing them is described. The results are then presented, discussed and summarised.

The quantitative part of the study sought to answer the following research question:

> How do nurses perceive spiritual need and spiritual care and profess to give it in practice?

This question was addressed by posing a number of sub-questions which guided the tool design. These are outlined below:

1   What do nurses understand by spiritual needs?

2   What do nurses understand by spiritual care?

3   Do nurses identify patients' spiritual needs?

4   How do nurses identify patients' spiritual needs?

5   How do nurses respond to patients' spiritual needs?

6   How do nurses evaluate the interventions employed to help patients meet their spiritual needs?

12 Method

Method and rationale for its selection

Recognising that every method has its strengths and weaknesses it was important to select the one most appropriate to the research questions. In this case a purpose designed postal questionnaire was chosen. The limitations of this method were acknowledged (Hoinville et al., 1978; Oppenheim, 1966; Polit and Hungler, 1987) and a variety of measures employed to minimise their effects as outlined in Table 1.

Despite these limitations, this method was considered the most appropriate for collecting data relevant to the research questions for the following reasons:

1   As nothing was known about how nurses perceived spiritual care it was considered important, initially, to gather this information from as many nurses as possible. As the population was distributed over a wide geographical area, the postal questionnaire was the only practical method available.

2   It was felt that more honest answers might be obtained as a consequence of respondents feeling less inhibited than may have been the case had an interviewer been present.

3   Because questions were standardised, responses would be free from interviewer bias and data would be relatively easy to process and analyse.

Table 4.1
Limitations of the postal questionnaire and measures employed to minimise them

Limitation	Measure(s) employed to minimise/ overcome it
1 The response rate achieved from questionnaires is usually lower than that of interviews.	The questionnaire and cover letter were designed in order to maximise the response rate, using recommendations given in the literature.
2 The researcher was totally dependent on the ability of respondents to interpret the questions correctly and complete the questionnaire according to the given instructions.	The questionnaire was carefully constructed and rigorously tested through the pre-pilots and the final pilot study. Changes were made in the light of the findings.
3 Factors which may have affected the validity of responses could not be controlled e.g., one had to trust that the answers given were those of the respondent and not someone else's.	Care was taken to ensure that each questionnaire was received by the nurse intended by enclosing it in a sealed envelope stating the nurse's name. If a nurse could not be traced, nurse managers were asked to return the questionnaire to the researcher. To encourage the nurse in receipt of the questionnaire to respond personally, the cover letter asked him/her not to collaborate with any one else while completing it.
4 There was no guarantee that the information provided by respondents was a true reflection of their practice.	Unfortunately little could be done about this and the researcher had to rely on a measure of honesty.
5 There was no guarantee that the information provided by respondents would be interpreted accurately by the researcher.	As people do not always answer questions under the given headings, the researcher sought to interpret the answer to each question in the context

Limitation	Measure(s) employed to minimise/ overcome it
	of each nurse's entire response. These interpretations would be checked with nurses selected for interview in Part 2 of the study. Reliability checks would be employed.
6 The researcher was dependent on the national and internal hospital mailing systems to ensure safe delivery of the questionnaires.	Although there was no viable way of checking that every questionnaire arrived at its intended destination, every hospital to which questionnaires had been sent was checked to see that at least one return had been received from it. In this way it was hoped that any gross failures in delivery would be highlighted.
7 The information obtained would be more superficial than that achieved using qualitative methods.	It was the intention that more in-depth information would be obtained in Part 2 of the study.

Source: Author's own

Design of the tool

Having decided to use a postal questionnaire this, together with a cover letter were designed and subjected to numerous pre-pilot tests before the final version emerged for use in the pilot study.

One of the major disadvantages of the postal questionnaire, acknowledged in Table 1, was that of poor response. This is often attributed to factors such as the subject under study, the population selected and sponsoring body, over which the researcher has little control, and to the limited means which exist, namely in the form of the cover letter, to encourage subjects to respond (Forcese and Richer, 1973). It was important, therefore, to encourage compliance by manipulating those factors under the researcher's control.

Thus the questionnaire and cover letter were designed, as described below, on the basis of guidelines taken from a variety of texts (Goode and Hatt, 1952; Gordon and Stokes, 1989; Moser and Kalton, 1971; Polit and Hungler, 1987).

The questionnaire

Six aspects were considered in designing the questionnaire as outlined below.

1 Questions included Care was taken to include only questions relevant to the study aims. The questionnaire was designed in three parts: A, B and C.

Part A: Because the literature review highlighted how personal characteristics of the nurse might influence the way in which they gave spiritual care, in order to explore this, Part A together with question 5 in Part B sought demographic information about respondents. Respondents were informed of the reason for obtaining this information.

Part B: All questions in Part B, with the exception of Q5, were included to determine how nurses perceived spiritual need and spiritual care and how they gave it in practice.

Part C: Part C was included to ascertain respondents' reasons, unforeseen by the researcher, for not wishing to complete the questionnaire and therefore to highlight possible characteristics of the non-respondent group.

2 Question wording and order Ambiguities and leading questions were avoided, abstract questions kept to a minimum and questions ordered logically, starting with the least threatening.

3 Question type Open, as well as closed questions were included to obtain more detailed information from respondents. Adequate space was provided for answers.

4 Question content In closed questions categories were mutually exclusive, the 'other' option was included and space for additional comments was provided.

5 Appearance Care was taken in the lay-out of the questionnaire e.g., spacing, type set. Additionally, as the literature suggested that colour of paper may have a bearing on the response rate, a mini-pilot study was conducted to ascertain the preferred colours, i.e., green and cream, both of which were used.

6 Practicalities Pre-paid envelopes were included and the study was launched before the summer holiday period.

The cover letter

Care was taken to ensure that the cover letter performed the following functions:

1 Provided respondents with information in relation to: the researcher; the subject and purpose of the enquiry; measures taken to ensure confidentiality; instructions for participation.

2 Encouraged nurses to respond by thanking them in advance and stressing the importance of their participation.

3 Gave credibility to the study by using a letter head and obtaining the support and approval of both the Head of Department where the researcher was based (by enclosing her signature) and the relevant authorities within the respondents' Health Authority/Board.

In an attempt to further increase the response rate, all letters were signed individually (Gordon and Stokes 1989) and kept as informal and short as possible.

The pilot study

Having designed the tool and carried out a number of pre-pilot tests, it was necessary to conduct a pilot study before launching the main study. This section outlines the reasons for doing so, the method used, the outcome and recommendations for change in the main study on the basis of the pilot work.

Purpose

The functions of the pilot study were to:

1 Test the questions contained within the questionnaire for ambiguities and ensure that they obtained the desired information.

2 Test the research method so that actual/potential problems could be identified and remedied before launching the main study.

3 Obtain some indication of: the length of time required for respondents to complete the questionnaire so that participants in the main study could be advised of this in advance.

4 Obtain an indication of the likely response rate for the main study.

Method

Selection of area and population Care was taken to ensure that the setting of and population for inclusion in the pilot study reflected that of the main study as closely as possible. Because it was intended to include every Health Board in Scotland in the main study, S/N's and C/N's for the pilot study were selected from a Health Authority in the north of England which contained 'care of the elderly' wards both within general and geriatric NHS hospitals.

Process for conducting the pilot study Hospitals containing 'care of the elderly' wards within the chosen Health Authority were identified (Chaplin, 1989). Permission to conduct the pilot study was sought from the appropriate authority and nurse managers were contacted to obtain their co-operation and the names of nurses for inclusion in the pilot study.

Questionnaires were sent, in individually labelled envelopes, to the nurse managers for distribution to the total population of nurses (n=15). Nurses were asked to return their completed forms to the researcher, within two weeks, using the pre-paid envelopes provided. As it was generally agreed in the literature that some form of reminder is usually required to boost the response rate (Goode and Hatt, 1952, Forcese and Richer, 1973, Kane, 1985, Polit and Hungler, 1987), a combined letter of thanks and reminder was sent to all nurses (to maintain confidentiality), via the nurse managers, three weeks after the initial mailing.

On receipt of the questionnaires, data were processed and analysed with the help of SPSS. Part of the analysis involved categorising responses to open questions. Because this gave rise to the possibility of researcher bias, a reliability check was carried out by comparing the categories produced by the researcher with those reached by two independent people who had been provided with the raw data. One person was a final year degree nursing student who had a particular interest in the subject under study and the other was a chartered accountant who had no connections with nursing.

The categories produced by both people were very similar to those of the researcher. Minor differences were noted in relation to the number of categories produced rather than the content. Thus from the small number of people who participated in the reliability check for the pilot study, researcher bias was not obvious. The categories are outlined in Table 4.3.

Outcome

The response rate to and the results of the pilot study are presented and briefly discussed.

Response rate   The response rate is shown in Table 4.2 below.

Table 4.2
Response rate of the pilot study

	No.	%
Total questionnaires sent out	15	100.0
Returns from initial mailing, before posting out of the reminder letter	4	26.7
Returns received following the mailing of the reminder letter	1	6.7
Total completed questionnaires received	5	33.3
Questionnaires returned uncompleted from nurse managers because respondent had left employment	1	6.7
Questionnaires not returned	9	60.0

Source: Author's own

The 33.3% (n=5) response rate was disappointing and less than satisfactory. The fact that nine out of fourteen nurses did not reply, even with the use of a reminder letter, was a matter for concern. One possible explanation was that subjects had been invited to participate in the pilot rather than the main study.

   It appeared, therefore, that additional measures would be required to increase the response rate in the main study as discussed later.

Results and discussion   The results of the pilot study are presented in Table 4.3. Because of the small numbers involved, percentages have been omitted.

   Little could be concluded from the results, given that only five usable questionnaires were returned. It is noteworthy, however, that all of those responding were C/N's with considerable experience, claiming some form of religious affiliation.

Table 4.3
Results of the pilot study

Part A of the questionnaire

	No. of nurses
Grade	
Charge nurse	5
Staff nurse	0
Sex	
Female	5
Male	0
Age	
< 21 years	0
21-29 years	0
30-39 years	1
40-49 years	2
50-59 years	2
60> years	0
Length of time in practice	
Less than 1 year	0
1-5 years	0
6-10 years	0
11-25 years	2
26 years and over	3
Type of ward	
Long term care	2
Geriatric rehabilitation	1
Combined long term care + geriatric rehabilitation	1
Combined long term care, geriatric rehabilitation + accident & emergency	1
Type of duty	
Day duty	4
Night duty	1
Rotation of day and night duty	0

Part B of the questionnaire

Nurses' definitions of spiritual need

1 Need for/of religion including: need to practise religious   1
  beliefs; need to turn/return to religious commitment.
2 Need of the 'soul'.   1
3 Need to talk to church member/nurse about individual needs.   1
4 Need for/of religion and need to feel that beliefs are respected   1
5 Needs of the 'inner self' and need for belief in something/someone.   1

Nurses' definitions of spiritual care

1 Take account of patients' beliefs/religious beliefs and help them   3
  with their customs whatever these may be.
2 As in 1 above and give the patient 'peace of mind'.   1
  Did not answer the question.   1

**Person nurses' stated they considered to be responsible for
responding to patients' spiritual needs**

1 Nurse alone.   0
2 Nurse and clergy.   4
3 Clergy alone.   0
4 No-one.   0
5 Anyone who can help.   1

**Nurses' statements of whether or not they had identified a
spiritual need**

1 Yes.   4
2 No.   1

**Indicators nurses stated they used in recognising
spiritual needs**

1 Patient's fear of death.   1
2 Unresponsiveness of patient.   1
3 Patient appeared distraught and afraid of death.   1
4 Patient talked about his/her faith.   1
5 Did not answer the question.   1

Nurses' stated responses to patients' spiritual needs

1 Talked with patient about their situation. Suggested contact/   3
  contacted clergy.
2 Contacted member of family to find out patient's religious needs.   1
3 Did not answer the question.   1

**Nurses' evaluations of the effectiveness of responses
made to patients' spiritual needs**

1 Totally effective.	1
2 More effective than ineffective.	2
3 Don't know.	1
4 More ineffective than effective.	0
5 Totally ineffective.	0
6 Did not answer the question.	1

**Factors nurses stated they used in evaluating the effectiveness
of their interventions**

1 Patient was more calm and returned to their 'old self'.	1
2 Patient was pleased to see clergy.	1
3 Complete/partial reduction of fear and acceptance of death indicated by ability to calmly and openly talk about it with staff and family.	1
4 Did not answer the question.	2

**Nurses' statements of whether or not they would have
responded any differently to patients' spiritual needs**

1 Yes.	0
2 No.	4
3 Did not answer the question.	1

**Ways in which nurses stated they would have responded
differently**

Did not answer the question.	5

Profession of religious affiliation

1 Yes.	5
2 No.	0

Type of religious affiliation claimed

1 Church of England.	4
2 Roman Catholic.	1

Part C of the questionnaire
Reasons given for not completing the questionnaire

Did not answer the question	5

Source: Author's own

It seemed that nurses tended to view spiritual need in religious terms and considered spiritual care to involve responding to these needs through formal religious means. Four of the five nurses said they had identified a spiritual need at some point in their practice, whether through some form of distress displayed by the patient or because the patient conveyed this verbally.

All five nurses considered it their duty to respond to patients' spiritual needs. Three of the four nurses who had identified a spiritual need responded by discussing this with the patient and then referring/suggesting referral to the clergy. One collaborated with the patient's family.

Three of the four nurses considered their action to have been effective because of eustressing (opposite of distress) characteristics observed in the patient. One was unsure of how effective her intervention had been.

Changes in the main study on the basis of the pilot study

No ambiguities were identified in the questions included in the questionnaire and the information sought was obtained.

Concerning the method, only minor alterations were made. Quotations from the codes of conduct were removed from the cover letter because some nurses responded using phrases similar to those quoted therein. Also the code numbers were transferred from the text to columns at the side of the questionnaire because the layout appeared to cause confusion.

Respondents in the pilot study indicated that they had taken 10-20 minutes to complete the questionnaire. This information was, therefore, included in the cover letter for the main study.

As previously discussed, additional measures would be required to boost the response rate in the main study. Having made the above amendments, the cover letter and questionnaire for the main study were finalised.

Operationalisation of the quantitative approach

Having completed the pilot study and made the necessary alterations, the main study was launched and conducted in accordance with the process outlined in Figure 4.1.

Response rate and problem of non-response

Having conducted the study according to the process outlined in Figure 4.1, 637 questionnaires (54.4%) were returned of which 529 (45.2%) were usable as illustrated in Table 4.4.

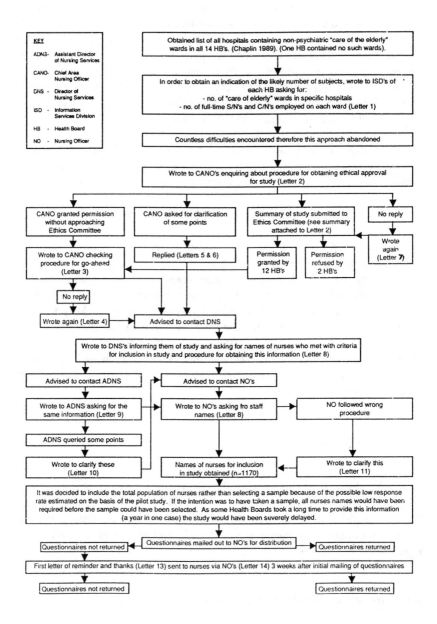

KEY

ADNS-	Assistant Director of Nursing Services
CANO-	Chief Area Nursing Officer
DNS -	Director of Nursing Services
ISD -	Information Services Division
HB -	Health Board
NO -	Nursing Officer

Obtained list of all hospitals containing non-psychiatric "care of the elderly" wards in all 14 HB's. (Chaplin 1989). (One HB contained no such wards).

In order to obtain an indication of the likely number of subjects, wrote to ISD's of each HB asking for:
- no. of "care of elderly" wards in specific hospitals
- no. of full-time S/N's and C/N's employed on each ward (Letter 1)

Countless difficulties encountered therefore this approach abandoned

Wrote to CANO's enquiring about procedure for obtaining ethical approval for study (Letter 2)

CANO granted permission without approaching Ethics Committee

CANO asked for clarification of some points

Summary of study submitted to Ethics Committee (see summary attached to Letter 2)

No reply

Wrote again (Letter 7)

Wrote to CANO checking procedure for go-ahead (Letter 3)

Replied (Letters 5 & 6)

Permission granted by 12 HB's

Permission refused by 2 HB's

No reply

Wrote again (Letter 4)

Advised to contact DNS

Wrote to DNS's informing them of study and asking for names of nurses who met with criteria for inclusion in study and procedure for obtaining this information (Letter 8)

Advised to contact ADNS

Advised to contact NO's

Wrote to ADNS asking for the same information (Letter 9)

Wrote to NO's asking fro staff names (Letter 8)

NO followed wrong procedure

ADNS queried some points

Wrote to clarify these (Letter 10)

Names of nurses for inclusion in study obtained (n=1170)

Wrote to clarify this (Letter 11)

It was decided to include the total population of nurses rather than selecting a sample because of the possible low response rate estimated on the basis of the pilot study. If the intention was to have taken a sample, all nurses names would have been required before the sample could have been selected. As some Health Boards took a long time to provide this information (a year in one case) the study would have been severely delayed.

Questionnaires not returned

Questionnaires mailed out to NO's for distribution

Questionnaires returned

First letter of reminder and thanks (Letter 13) sent to nurses via NO's (Letter 14) 3 weeks after initial mailing of questionnaires

Questionnaires not returned

Questionnaires returned

Figure 4.1 Operationalisation of the quantitative approach
Source   Author's own

Table 4.4
Initial response rate to the main study

	No.	%
Total questionnaires sent out.	1170	100.0
Questionnaires returned from initial mailing before posting out of Reminder Letter 1.	372	31.8
Questionnaires returned following mailing of Reminder Reminder Letter 1.	157	13.4
Questionnaires returned but unusable because respondents did not meet with criteria for the study.	34	2.9
Questionnaires returned uncompleted from nurse managers.	74	6.3
Total questionnaires returned.	637	54.4
Usable questionnaires.	529	52.0
Questionnaires not returned.	533	45.6

Source: Author's own

The response rate of 54.4% achieved in the main study was higher than that expected (i.e., 30-35% from the pilot study). This may have been because respondents valued participation in the main study more highly than the pilot study. The necessity of employing additional measures to increase the response rate, as recommended by the pilot study, was therefore questioned and the literature was reviewed to see what was an acceptable response rate. Response rates from as low as 0% (Ferber, 1948 in Robin, 1973) to as high as over 90% (Moser and Kalton, 1971) were reported. However, there appeared to be a consensus of opinion that a 40-60% response rate was 'good' (Bailey, 1978 in Kane, 1985, Oppenheim, 1966, Orenstein and Phillips, 1978, Warwick and Lininger, 1975) with that in excess of 75% being exceptional (Goode and Hatt, 1952 in Robin, 1973, Oppenheim, 1966, Warwick and Lininger, 1975).

According to the literature, therefore, the 54.4% response rate achieved in this study was acceptable. However, this still meant that almost half (45.6%) of the nurses had failed to respond. The researcher was concerned that those who had responded perhaps held different views on the subject under study from those who had not responded and were, therefore, unrepresentative of the total population of nurses (Robin, 1973, Youngman, 1978). For instance it was suspected that some nurses may not have responded due to lack of time or interest in the subject (Moser and Kalton, 1971) especially if they held more neutral opinions on spiritual care (Boek and Laid, 1963, Katz and Cantril, 1937, Franzen and Lazersfeld, 1945 all in Champion and Sear, 1973).

As Oppenheim (1966, p.34) states:

Non-response it not a random process, but has its own determinants.

In spite of the literature, therefore, in order to minimise the effects of possible non-respondent bias, it was decided to employ measures to increase the response rate further by sending a second reminder letter and copy of the questionnaire to the non-respondent group (Forcese and Richer, 1973, Moser and Kalton, 1971, Youngman, 1978).

Before this was done, however, some assurance that such an intervention would be economically viable was sought.

Using the rough guideline that:

something like the same proportion of persons sent questionnaires respond to each mailing (Moser and Kalton, 1971, p.266)

it was estimated that, of the non-respondent group (n=533), 31.8% (Table 4.4) would respond to the second mailing resulting in an additional 170 questionnaires being received. This would increase the overall response rate by 14.5%.

Using the above estimate, it was decided to check the effectiveness of the second mailing by sending a second reminder letter and questionnaire to non-respondents in one randomly selected Health Board. As the response rate was higher (42%) than expected (33.4%), this procedure was repeated in all other Health Boards. In total, 156 additional questionnaires were received raising the overall response rate of the study by 13.3% to 67.8% as shown in Table 4.5.

Table 4.5
Response rate to the main study

	No.	%
Questionnaires returned following mailing of the second reminder letter and second copy of the questionnaire.	156	13.3
Total questionnaires returned.	793	67.8
Total usable questionnaires.	685	58.5
Total questionnaires not returned.	377	32.2

Source: Author's own

Data processing

As both closed and open questions were included in the questionnaire, responses to each required a different method of processing. Both of these methods, together with details of a reliability check employed, are described in this section.

Processing of responses to closed questions

Closed questions included all questions in Part A of the questionnaire and questions 3,4.1, 4.4a, 4.5, 5 in Part B.
    Responses to these questions were processed as described below.
    All responses were allocated code numbers which were inserted in the 'code' column of the questionnaire.
    Responses to questions containing the 'other' option, (i.e., Part A question 4 and Part B questions 3 and 5b), were allocated to categories which emerged directly from the data. These are outlined in Figures 4.9, 4.13 and Table 4.9. The appropriate code numbers were then entered in the 'code' column of the questionnaires.
    All codes were entered into the SPSS data file.

Processing of responses to open questions

Open questions included questions 1, 2, 4.2, 4.3, 4.4b, 4.6 in Part B of the questionnaire and Part C.

The 'Ethnograph' package was used to assist in the processing of responses to open questions. This package was developed by American social scientists (Seidel et al., 1988) who were involved in qualitative research and was designed to assist with the analysis of text based data. It enables the researcher to code, recode and sort data into categories. Sections of text can then be displayed, sorted and printed in any order. It is important to note that the programme only acts as a mechanical aid. It does not take over any of the thinking aspects of the analysis. Rather, by performing the time consuming tasks of 'cutting and pasting', which was previously a laborious part of a qualitative researcher's work, it releases the researcher to devote time to the more crucial interpretative analysis. In this way the Ethnograph proved invaluable to the researcher in managing data relevant to open questions.

Responses to each open question were assigned to categories which emerged from the data. New categories were created only when responses could not be classified under previously established categories. Because questions 2 and 4.3 in Part B of the questionnaire seemed to elicit similar information, they were combined and treated as a single question.

Initially the number of categories per question was very large e.g., 70 for one question, therefore all categories were collapsed.

Given the large number of categories still existing, some of which contained few responses, it was decided to merge categories where common themes existed.

In doing so it was found that many new categories were similar to those identified in the literature. To detect researcher bias in the collapse of categories, the process by which this had occurred was checked independently by the project supervisors who were generally in agreement with the alterations made. The process is described below.

Merging of categories The way in which the categories relevant to each question in Part B and C of the questionnaire were merged is described in turn. Where similar categories had been identified in the literature, the relevant authors are stated.

Q1 How would you define the term 'spiritual need'?

Six new categories were produced from the original fifteen. These were:

1   Need for meaning, purpose and fulfilment. (Category similar to that identified by: Chomicz, 1984, Conrad 1985, Fish and Shelly, 1978, Highfield and Cason, 1983, Renetzky, 1979, Simsen, 1985, Stallwood-Hess, 1969). Collapsed under this category were:

'Need to find meaning in life' because it was directly relevant.

'Need to be alone/for reflection'. One of the indicators of the need for meaning and purpose identified by Highfield and Cason (1983) was 'exhibits emotional detachment from self and peers'. This suggests a desire to be alone. Furthermore the act of reflection is often closely associated with the search for meaning.

'Need for a sense of fulfilment/satisfaction'. Another indicator of the need for meaning cited in the study by Highfield and Cason (1983) was 'expresses contentment'. According to the dictionary (Macdonald, 1972), contentment and satisfaction are synonymous. Furthermore Renetzky (1979) classes the need for fulfilment together with the need for meaning and purpose.

2   Need to give and receive love and forgiveness. (Category similar to that identified by: Chance, 1967, Chomicz, 1984, Conrad, 1985, Fish and Shelly, 1978, Highfield and Cason, 1983, Jacik, 1989, Simsen, 1985, Stallwood-Hess, 1969). Collapsed under this category were:

'Need for love, unity and forgiveness' because it was of direct relevance.

'Need to talk about/explore issues'. Although this would also have fitted under the 'need for meaning, purpose and fulfilment', it was decided to place it here because two of the indicators of the need for love and forgiveness noted by Highfield and Cason (1983) were : 'does not discuss feelings about dying with significant others'; 'confesses thoughts and feelings about which he is ashamed'. Central to the above statements is talking and exploring.

3   Need for hope and creativity. (Category similar to that identified by: Chance, 1967, Chomicz ,1984, Conrad, 1985, Highfield and Cason, 1983, Renetzky, 1979, Simsen, 1985). Included in this category were:

'Need for a sense of elation/joy/exuberance/more of life'. Two of the indicators of the need for hope and creativity mentioned by Highfield and Cason (1983) were 'boredom' and 'unable to pursue creative outlets'. The experience of elation etc., seemed to represent the opposite end of the spectrum for these expressions. In addition the need for the will to live, which is similar to the desire for more of life, was a spiritual need identified by Renetzky (1979) and is closely linked with hope.

'Need for hope' because it was directly relevant.

4 Need for belief and faith. (Category similar to that identified by Chance, 1967, Chomicz, 1984, Renetzky, 1979, Simsen, 1985). Included in this category was 'Need to believe in something/someone' because it was obviously connected.

5 Need for peace and comfort. (Category similar to that identified by Jacik, 1989). Included in this category were:

'Need to achieve a state of comfort' because it was of direct relevance.

'Need which appears in crisis and, in particular, on approaching death'. Only when an individual has come to terms with a situation e.g., death, can they experience a sense of peace and comfort.

6 Miscellaneous. Included in this category were:

'A need which is more than: physical; mental; emotional; social'.

'A psychological or emotional need'.

'A deep inner need. A need of the soul or core of the person'.

'An individual need which varies from person to person'.

'With difficulty'.

None of the above fitted any of the previous five categories or was mentioned often enough to warrant a separate category.

Q2 How would you define the term 'spiritual care'? and Q4.3 What did you do in response to this need?

1 Recognising/respecting/meeting patients spiritual needs.(Category similar to that identified by Stallwood-Hess 1969). Included in this category were:

'Recognising/respecting/meeting patients' spiritual needs' because it obviously fits.

'Did nothing. Respected patient's wishes for no action to be taken' because by taking no action the nurse was showing respect.

'Finding out more about patients' beliefs'. It was assumed that the nurse was attempting to find out more about the patient's beliefs so that care could be given to the patient in a manner which was in keeping with those beliefs.

'Documenting nursing process records'. In doing this it was assumed that the nurse was ensuring continuity of care in keeping with their beliefs.

2 Facilitating participation in religious rituals. (Category similar to that identified by Carson, 1989, Chance, 1967, Martin et al., 1976, Stallwood-Hess, 1969). Included was 'Enabling patients to meet their spiritual needs' because all activities to which this statement refers were concerned with helping patients perform religious acts.

3 Communicating: listening; talking with. (Category similar to that identified by Carson, 1989, Chance, 1967, Martin et al., 1976, Stallwood-Hess, 1969). Included were:

'Communicating with patients/relatives' because all the items included under this heading involved talking, exploring, guiding and listening, all of which are modes of communication.

'Using humour' because the essence in which humour was used was in guiding the patient toward reality and acceptance of the situation they were in.

'Distracting the patient from the present situation' for the same reason as given for 'using humour'.

4 Being with the patient: caring, supporting, showing empathy. (Category similar to that identified by Carson, 1989, Martin et al., 1976). Included were:

'Caring for and supporting the patient/family'.

'Giving/sharing of self'.

'Being there'.

'Supporting the patient'.

All of the above clearly corresponded with the category description.

5 Promoting a sense of well-being. Although this was not a category found in any previous studies it emerged directly from the data and was felt to be significantly different from all other categories to warrant separate attention. Included were:

'Promoting a sense of well-being' as it was of obvious relevance.

'Helping the patient generally'. By generally helping and carrying out patients' requests/wishes the nurse can promote a sense of well-being by making the patient feel worthwhile.

'Giving the patient self esteem'. By catering to the patient's esteem needs a sense of well-being can be facilitated.

6 Referring to others (Category similar to that identified by Carson, 1989, Chance, 1967, Martin et al., 1976, Stallwood-Hess, 1969). Included was 'Referring to others' as all items included under this heading involved referral whether directly or indirectly.

7 Expressed difficulty in defining or giving spiritual care. Included was 'Expressed difficulty in defining or giving spiritual care' because it obviously fitted.

Q4.2 How did you recognise this need?

The number of categories was reduced from 11 to six as outlined below. Few studies addressed the issue of indicators of spiritual need, the main one being that of Chance (1967). Highfield and Cason (1983) cited many indicators of spiritual need but they did not categorise these.

1 The need was expressed by the patient verbally or non-verbally. Included was 'through communication' because the central theme is the patient communicating their need through verbal or non-verbal means. Both modes of communication were mentioned by Chance (1967).

2 The need was observed by the nurse in other ways. Included were:

'Through observation of the patient' because in all items included the spiritual need was detected through the nurse's observation of the patient.

'By knowing the patient' because it was through knowing/knowing something about the patient that the need was observed by the nurse.

3   Through distress displayed by the patient. Included were:

'Distress displayed by the patient' because it was of direct relevance. Chance (1967) also produced two categories namely 'emotional attitudes' and 'tears' which are similar to some aspects of this category.

'Patient was awkward/hostile'. The central theme was that of distress. Many of the characteristics outlined in this category were similarly identified by Highfield and Cason (1983) as indicators of spiritual distress.

'Physical signs'. The presence of pain, elevated blood pressure and pulse and failure of physical interventions to alleviate the problem can all either cause distress or indicate that the patient is distressed.

4   Through state of helplessness displayed by the patient. Included were:

'Helplessness'. Seligman's (1975) state of 'learned helplessness' seemed to best describe these characteristics identified by nurses as indicative of spiritual need. All involve one or more of the symptoms of this condition namely: passivity; negative cognitive set; lack of aggression; social deficits. The important distinction between this category and that of 'Distress' is that of apathy. In the 'Distress' category most of the characteristics are active e.g., anger, fear, aggression. Here there are no active states. Many of these characteristics were also identified by Highfield and Cason (1983).

'Low self esteem'. Vulnerability and unworthiness are themes alluded to by Seligman (1975) in his writings on learned helplessness.

5   Through patient's desire/inability to come to terms with situation. This category emerged directly from the data and was felt to be significantly different from all other categories to warrant separate attention. Included was:

'expressed desire/inability to come to terms with past/present/future' because it was directly relevant.

6   Positive characteristics displayed by the patient. All of the previously mentioned categories major on negative characteristics displayed by the patient. It was felt that the positive characteristics patients displayed which enabled nurses to recognise a spiritual need should be grouped together in the form of a separate category. Included were 'desire for life' and 'prepared for death' both being positive characteristics.

Q4.4b How effective do you consider this response was? What made you think that?

The number of categories was reduced from 10 to seven. Most of the indicators nurses stated had enabled them to evaluate the effectiveness of their interventions in meeting patients' spiritual needs were the opposite of those which had led them to identify the need initially. These are described below.

1   Eustressing characteristics displayed by the patient. Seleye's state of 'eustress', being the opposite of distress, seemed to best describe the characteristics mentioned in 'patient reached a state of eustress'.

2   Patient appeared brighter in mood. All of the characteristics outlined in the following categories opposed the state of helplessness/hopelessness.

     'Brighter in mood'.

     'Increased/improved relationships with others.

     'Increased self esteem'.

3   Patient's ability to accept situation. This was the opposite of 'inability to accept situation' mentioned in QB4.2. Included was 'able to accept or displayed signs of working towards acceptance of situation'.

4   Patient confirmed that his/her need had been met. The patient confirmed the above in the same ways that he/she had expressed the need in 'patient expressed the need' in QB4.2 i.e., using verbal and non-verbal communication. Included was 'confirmed by the patient in some way'.

5   Nurse felt the need was met. Not necessarily confirmed by the patient. The nurse observed that the need had been met in the same way that she had identified it in QB4.2 'Through observing the patient'. The emphasis is on observation and 'sensing'. Included was 'need had been met'.

6   Nurse felt that the need was not met/not completely met. In some instances, usually when they stated that their interventions had been ineffective, nurses felt that the patient's need had not been met. It was felt that the negative characteristics indicative of this should occupy a separate category. Included were:

     'Need was not met/not completely met'.

'Nurse felt inadequate in dealing with the situation'.

7 Nurse expressed difficulty in assessing the effectiveness of her interventions. Again it was felt that this group of responses was significantly different from all others to merit occupation of a separate category. Included was 'nurse did not know/found it difficult to assess the effectiveness of her response'.

Q4.6 What would you have done differently?

Given the small number of nurses who answered this question it proved difficult to reduce the categories further. Only two categories were collapsed namely:

1 'Involved others'.

2 'Tried to overcome own feeling of inadequacy'.

These were merged to form one category 'involved others/sought help' as it was assumed that in some cases nurses would have involved others because they felt unable or inadequate to deal with the situation.

Because of the small number of nurses who used Section C of the questionnaire, it was not possible to reduce the categories any further, therefore, they remain as listed in Table 4.16.

Reliability check

Having processed the data relevant to open questions, before they were entered into the SPSS data file for analysis, it was considered important to check that all the intended changes in the various categorisations of responses had been made correctly. Thus a reliability check was conducted on the 'Ethnograph' package and the researcher before questionnaires were checked generally for meaning. Each check is described in turn.

Checking the 'Ethnograph' package for reliability Every tenth intended change in categorisation was checked to make sure it had been made. Out of the 430 checks no errors were found as shown in the working below. (Formulae were obtained from Walsh, 1990).

$$\% \text{ error } = \frac{\text{number of errors}}{\text{total checks}} \times \frac{100}{1}$$

$$= \frac{0}{430} \times \frac{100}{1}$$

$$= 0$$

As the percentage error was zero, with any size of confidence limit it can be predicted that out of the total number of changes made by the 'Ethnograph' package, the % of errors will also be 0.

It was concluded, therefore, that the 'Ethnograph' package was a reliable tool.

Checking the reliability of the researcher   It was considered that researcher error would most likely arise from typing mistakes e.g., mis-spelling and inadvertent omission of code words. To check for this, for every question, a Health Board was chosen at random and the original codes intended for re-coding were re-typed into the computer. If all code words had been typed properly the first time all changes should have been made, therefore no changes should have occurred on the second typing (assuming that the second typing was correct).

Out of the 246 words re-typed, four typing errors were found. All errors were due to the researcher having failed to type some words rather than having typed the wrong words. All errors would have been detected in the final coding of responses because these particular code words were no longer in existence. The % of error found in the sample of words re-typed was 1.63% as shown in the following working:

$$\% \text{ error (p)} = \frac{\text{number of errors}}{\text{total checks}} \times \frac{100}{1}$$

$$= \frac{4}{246} \times \frac{100}{1}$$

$$= 1.63\%$$

Extending this to the total number of words typed, there was a 95% probability that the % of error lay between 0.048% and 3.21% as shown in the following working:

$$\text{Standard Error (SE) in the sample} = \sqrt{\frac{p(100-p)}{N}} \qquad p = \% \text{ of error in the sample}$$

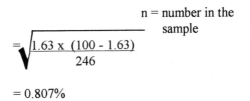

$$= \sqrt{\frac{1.63 \times (100 - 1.63)}{246}}$$

n = number in the sample

$$= 0.807\%$$

Using a 95% confidence interval, the % error estimated in the total words typed $= p \pm 1.96 \times SEp$

$$= 1.63 \pm 1.96 \times 0.807$$

$$= 0.048\% \text{ and } 3.21\%$$

It was concluded that the researcher was reliable in typing accurately. It was assumed, therefore, that the intended code words for change were altered correctly in the majority of instances. Given that the % error in the sample was negligible and that all would have been detected in the final check, it was not considered necessary to conduct a second check on all words typed.

Checking questionnaires for meaning As responses had been subjected to considerable re-coding, it was feared that the meaning of some responses may have been lost. Every tenth questionnaire (i.e., 63) was, therefore, checked by the researcher only to ensure that the meaning of each response was most appropriately captured by the category to which it had been assigned.

Out of the 468 code words checked from the 63 questionnaires, 68 errors were found. An error was considered to have occurred when a response which had been assigned to a category could, in the opinion of the researcher, have been more appropriately categorised.

The % error in the above sample was 14.53% as shown in the working below:

% error = $\frac{\text{number of errors}}{\text{total checks}} \times \frac{100}{1}$

$$= \frac{68}{468} \times \frac{100}{1}$$

$$= 14.53\%$$

As the next working illustrates there was a 95% probability that the % of errors in the total number of questionnaires lay between 11.33% and 17.72%:

$$SE = \sqrt{\frac{p\,(100 - p)}{N}}$$

$$= \sqrt{\frac{14.53 \times (100 - 14.53)}{468}}$$

$$= 1.63\%$$

Using a 95% confidence interval:

the % error $= p \pm 1.96 \times SEp$

$$= 14.53 \pm 3.194$$

$$= 11.33\% \text{ and } 17.72\%$$

It was felt that this incidence of error was too high, therefore all categorisations of responses in all questionnaires were re-checked for meaning and altered accordingly.

Data analysis

Having processed the data, they were analysed as follows.

1 Frequency distributions were conducted within SPSS to obtain demographic information and to ascertain how nurses perceived spiritual need and spiritual care and how they reported to have given it in practice.

2 In order to identify factors which appeared to influence the spiritual care given, a twofold approach was adopted.

First, factors reported by some nurses to have influenced the spiritual care given were noted.

Second, in order to more reliably identify factors which may have influenced the spiritual care given, variables were cross-tabulated in SPSS.

Cross-tabulation made it possible to establish if associations existed between variables and, if so, the probability that these associations could have occurred by chance. It was, however, not possible to determine the direction of the association or to prove cause and effect (Norusis, 1988; Reid and Boore, 1987).

The following section reports the results of these analyses.

13 Presentation and discussion of results

Having processed and analysed the data as outlined, the results are described and discussed in three sections. First the demographic data are presented. Second, nurses' perceptions of spiritual need and spiritual care and their reports of how they gave this are described and finally attention focuses on factors which appeared to be associated with the giving of spiritual care.

Demographic information about respondents

The demographic data, obtained from Part A and Part B Q5 of the questionnaire, are presented in a series of figures and the main points are highlighted. The following key outlines the abbreviations used for Health Boards.

Key for Health Boards

A&C	Argyll & Clyde
Bord	Borders
D&G	Dumfries & Galloway
F.V	Forth Valley
Gram	Grampian
Gt.G	Greater Glasgow
High	Highland
Lan	Lanarkshire
Loth	Lothian
Shet	Shetland
Tay	Tayside
W.I	Western Isles

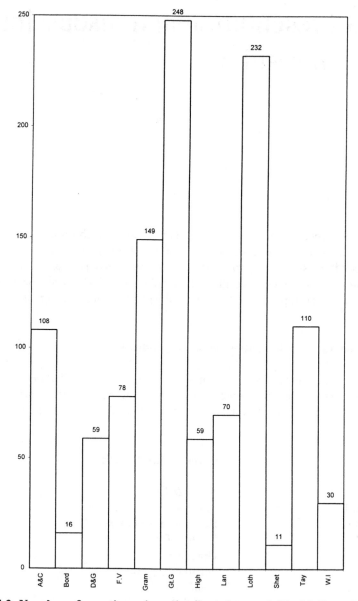

Figure 4.2 Number of questionnaires distributed to each Health Board
Source: Author's own

As Figure 4.2 shows, the number of questionnaires distributed to Health Boards was roughly in proportion to their size in terms of population.

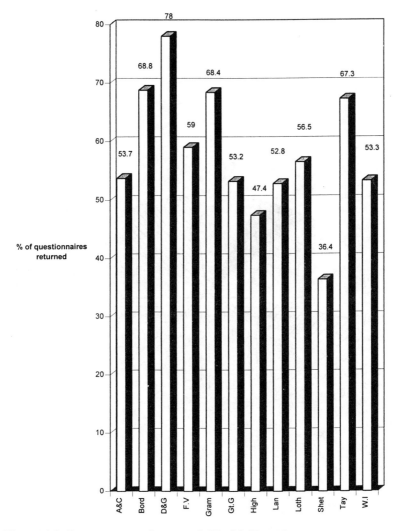

Figure 4.3 Response rate from each Health Board
Source: Author's own

The highest response rates were obtained from Dumfries and Galloway, Borders and Grampian (in descending order) and the lowest from Shetland, Highland and Lanarkshire (in ascending order). No clear explanation for this finding could be identified.

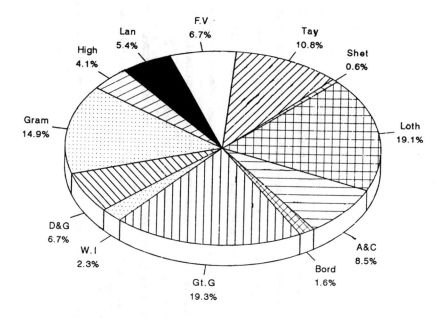

Figure 4.4 Distribution of respondents according to Health Board area
Source: Author's own

The distribution of respondents was roughly in proportion to Health Board
size in terms of population.

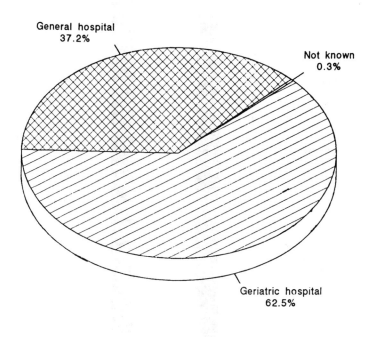

General hospital
37.2%

Not known
0.3%

Geriatric hospital
62.5%

Figure 4.5 Distribution of respondents according to hospital type
Source: Author's own

The majority of respondents were working in geriatric hospitals which was a reflection of the population distribution according to hospital type.   In two cases it was not known what type of hospital the nurses were working in as a nurse manager had photocopied questionnaires for these nurses thus the coding was lost.

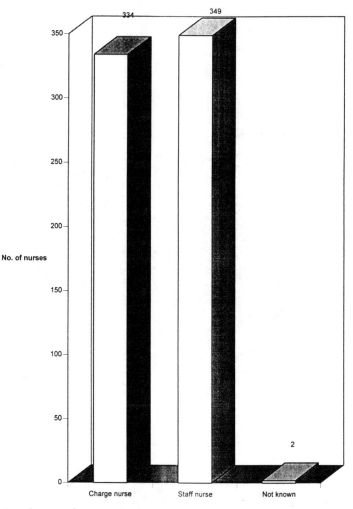

Figure 4.6 Grade of respondents
Source: Author's own

The highest proportion of respondents were S/N's, however, a higher percentage of C/N's responded than S/N's. The reason for this was not clear. However, it may have been that C/N's felt a greater obligation to respond because they had more personal contact with nurse managers who had distributed the questionnaires or because of their sense of overall managerial responsibility for patient care.

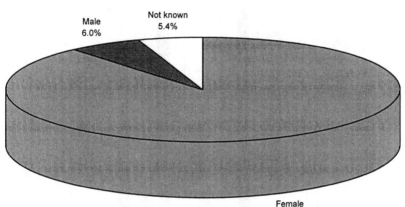

Male
6.0%

Not known
5.4%

Female
88.6%

Figure 4.7 Sex of respondents
Source: Author's own

As expected the majority of nurses were female.

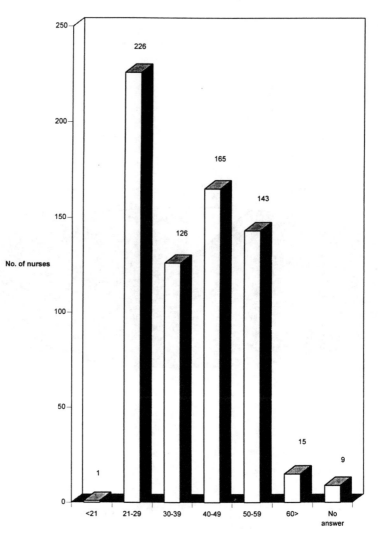

Figure 4.8 Age of respondents
Source: Author's own

The highest and lowest proportions of nurses responding were aged 21-29 years and under 21 years respectively. This distribution of respondents by age may reflect the proportion of nurses from each age group currently in practice, possible reasons for which are outlined in Table 4.6 below.

Table 4.6
Possible reasons for the proportion of nurses within each age group currently in practice

Age group	Possible reason
<21 years	Majority of S/N's are least 21 when qualified.
21-29 years	Upsurge of newly qualified S/N's.
30-39 years	A drop in numbers due to break in service for child rearing.
40-49 years	A slight increase in numbers as women return to work when children are older.
50-59 years	A slight drop in numbers as some nurses take early retirement or are promoted to more senior administrative posts.
60> years	A sharp drop in numbers due to retirement.

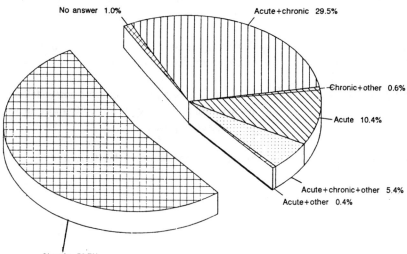

No answer 1.0% Acute+chronic 29.5%

Chronic+other 0.6%

Acute 10.4%

Acute+chronic+other 5.4%
Acute+other 0.4%

Chronic 52.7%

Figure 4.9 Distribution of respondents according to ward type
Source: Author's own

'Other' refers to any ward outwith care of the elderly e.g., medical, surgical, thoracic.

The majority of nurses were working on long term care of the elderly wards only (chronic) reflecting of the increasing elderly population in Britain and the predominance of this type of ward in geriatric hospitals where most respondents were situated.

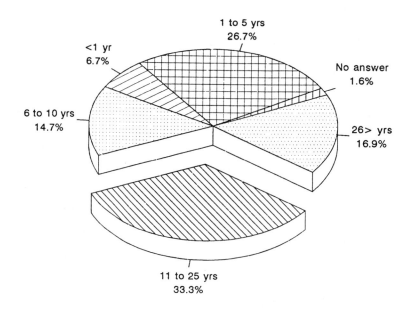

Figure 4.10 Length of time respondents had been in practice
Source: Author's own

The length of time respondents had been in practice is probably a reflection of their age. The highest proportion had been in practice 11-25 years and probably reflects the fact that this group could consist of nurses 30 years and over of which there are a substantial number (Figure 4.8) and can probably be explained by the reasons outlined in Table 4.6 for the <21, 21-29 and 50-60 year age groups.

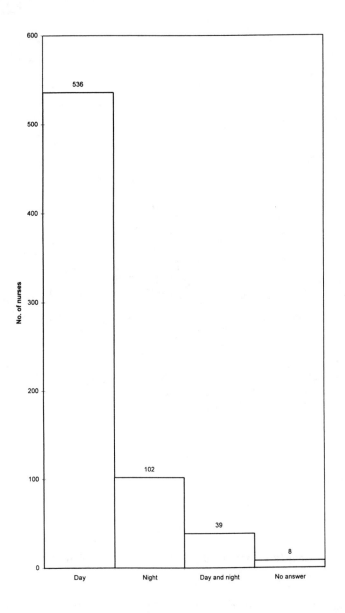

Figure 4.11 Distribution of respondents according to type of duty
Source: Author's own

The majority of nurses (536) were working day duty.

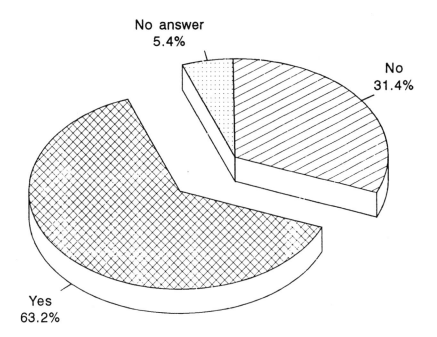

No answer
5.4%

No
31.4%

Yes
63.2%

Figure 4.12 Religious affiliation claimed by respondents
Source: Author's own

The majority of nurses claimed to possess some type of religious affiliation.
This may be explained by the fact that the majority of people, even if they have
merely had nominal church connections, e.g., have been christened, would
adopt some religious label.

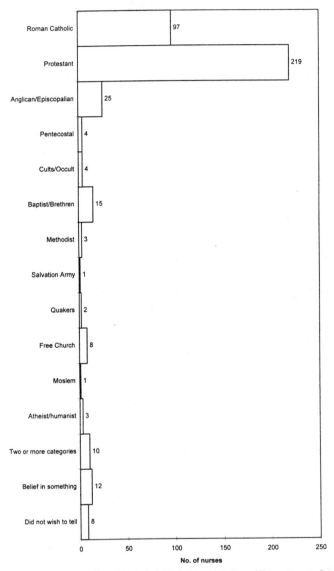

Figure 4.13 Type of religious affiliation claimed by respondents
Source: Author's own

Of those claiming religious affiliation (n=433), the majority (53.2%) described themselves as protestant, e.g., Church of Scotland, Presbyterian, Congregational, with smaller percentages classifying themselves as Roman Catholic (23.5%) and Anglican/Episcopalian (6.1%).

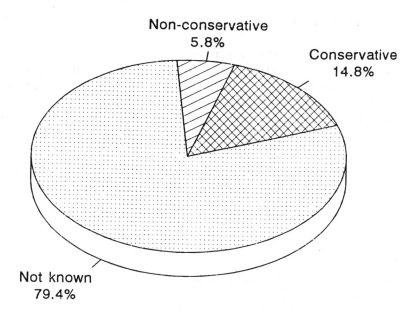

Non-conservative
5.8%

Conservative
14.8%

Not known
79.4%

Figure 4.14 Conservatism of belief of respondents
Source: Author's own

As it was thought that nurses who were conservative in their belief might view
and respond differently to spiritual needs than those with no/nominal religious
belief, where possible this distinction was made. Unfortunately, in the majority
of cases, it was not possible to ascertain this information therefore any analyses
conducted using this variable were limited.

Nurses' perceptions of spiritual need and care and their reports of how they gave this care

In this section nurses' perceptions of spiritual need and spiritual care and how they reported to have given this care are presented and discussed before conclusions are drawn.

Presentation of results

The results are presented in a series of tables.

The tables are ordered according to the sequence in which questions appeared in the questionnaire. As previously outlined, questions B2 and 4.3 were combined.

Throughout, percentages are expressed in terms of the total number of respondents who answered the particular question.

Table 4.7
Nurses' definitions of spiritual need

Definition	No and % of nurses giving each response	
	No.	%
1 Need for meaning, purpose and fulfilment.	64	9.9
2 Need to give and receive love and forgiveness.	91	14.1
3 Need for hope and creativity.	23	3.6
4 Need for belief and faith.	221	34.1
5 Need for peace and comfort.	158	24.4
6 Miscellaneous.	90	3.9
7 Did not answer the question.	38	

Table 4.8
Nurses' definitions of spiritual care and/or stated responses to patients' spiritual needs

Definition/response	No and % of nurses giving each response	
	No.	%
1 Recognising/respecting/meeting patients' spiritual needs.	44	6.8
2 Facilitating participation in religious rituals.	43	6.7
3 Communicating: listening/talking with.	42	6.5
4 Being with the patient: caring, supporting, showing empathy.	121	18.8
5 Promoting a sense of well-being.	58	9.0
6 Referring to others.	333	51.6
7 Expressed difficulty in defining or giving spiritual care.	4	0.6
8 Did not answer the question.	40	

Table 4.9
People nurses considered to be responsible for responding to patients' spiritual needs

Person	No and % of nurses giving each response	
	No.	%
1 Nurse alone.	0	0.0
2 Clergy alone.	37	5.6
3 No-one.	2	0.3
4 Nurse and clergy.	485	73.5
5 *Other (Only in 0.4% of cases did nurses exclude themselves from this role).	136	20.6
6 Did not answer the question.	25	

* Includes any combination of the following: anyone; those outwith the health care team, e.g., family and friends; clergy and those outwith the health care team; nurse and clergy and those outwith the health care team.

Table 4.10
Nurses' reports of whether or not they had identified a spiritual need

Had identified a spiritual need	No and % of nurses giving each response	
	No.	%
1 Yes.	503	76.8
2 No.	152	23.2
3 Did not answer the question.	30	

Table 4.11
Indicators nurses stated they used in recognising patients' spiritual needs

Indicators	No and % of nurses giving each response	
	No.	%
1 The need was expressed by the patient verbally or non-verbally.	155	31.4
2 The need was observed in other ways by by the nurse.	111	22.5
3 Through distress displayed by the patient.	125	25.3
4 Through state of helplessness displayed by the patient.	47	9.5
5 Through patient's inability to come to terms with situation.	49	9.9
6 Positive characteristics displayed by the patient.	7	1.4
7 Did not answer the question.	191	

Table 4.12
Nurses' evaluations of the effectiveness of responses to patients' spiritual needs

Efficacy	No and % of nurses giving each response	
	No.	%
1 Totally effective.	146	29.2
2 More effective than ineffective.	276	55.2
3 Don't know	55	11.0
4 More ineffective than effective.	17	3.4
5 Totally ineffective.	6	1.2
6 Did not answer the question.	185	

Table 4.13
Indicators nurses stated they used in evaluating the effectiveness of responses to patients' spiritual needs

Indicators	No and % of nurses giving each response	
	No.	%
1 Eustressing characteristics displayed by the patient.	174	37.6
2 Patient appeared brighter in mood.	48	10.4
3 Patient's ability to accept situation.	35	7.6
4 Patient confirmed that his/her need had been met.	78	16.8
5 Nurse felt that the need had been met. Not necessarily confirmed by the patient.	46	9.9
6 Nurse felt that the need was not met/not completely met.	28	8.0
7 Nurse expressed difficulty is assessing the effectiveness of his/her interventions.	54	9.7
8 Did not answer the question.	222	

Source: Tables 4.7 to 4.13 author's own reproduced by kind permission of
Blackwell Science Ltd. from Ross (1994)

Table 4.14
Nurses' statements of whether or not they would have responded differently to patients' spiritual needs

Would have responded differently	No and % of nurses giving each response	
	No.	%
1 Yes.	50	10.1
2 No.	443	89.5
3 Don't know.	2	0.4
4 Did not answer the question.	190	

Source: Author's own

Table 4.15
Ways in which nurses stated they would have responded differently

Alternative responses	No and % of nurses giving each response	
	No.	%
1 Acted earlier.	3	6.7
2 Spent more time with patient/family.	12	26.7
3 Involved others/sought help.	23	51.1
4 Included spiritual care in the nursing process.	4	8.9
5 Prayed with patient.	3	6.7
6 Did not answer the question.	640	

Source: Author's own

Table 4.16
Reasons for nurses not completing the questionnaire

Reasons	No and % of nurses giving each response	
	No.	%
1 Very private and personal thing.	4	18.1
2 Did not feel able to participate.	4	8.1
3 Spiritual care should be left to the chaplain.	3	13.6
4 No time.	1	4.6
5 Would have preferred to have been invited to respond.	1	4.6
6 Did not feel qualified to give spiritual care.	4	18.1
7 Found questions difficult to answer.	2	9.1
8 Working with the confused elderly who are unable to express spiritual needs.	1	4.6
9 Have not encountered anyone with a spiritual need.	1	4.6
10 Did not feel that the subject could be generalised.	1	4.6
11 Did not answer the question.	663	

Source: Author's own

Discussion of results

This section consists of three parts. First the results are discussed in general terms. Second they are compared with findings in other studies. Third the main findings are summarised.

General discussion of results As discussed in Part 2, the nursing process was suggested as the framework within which spiritual care could be given. Nurses' perceptions of spiritual need, spiritual care and their reports of how they gave this care are, therefore, discussed in accordance with the stages of the nursing process. In addition the reasons nurses gave for not completing the questionnaire are considered. Reference is made throughout the discussion to the relevant tables in the results section. Unless otherwise stated, the discussion centres on the 685 responses received.

Assessment In general it seemed that nurses had identified patients' spiritual needs, as indicated by the fact that the majority (76.8%) claimed to have done so (Table 4.10), however it was not possible to determine the extent to which they had identified these needs.

This still meant that 152 nurses (23.2%) had never identified a spiritual need in any patients at any point in their practice. It may have been that none of the patients these nurses looked after had spiritual needs, however, some of them may have done. For those patients who had spiritual needs the implication is that, unless their needs were identified by someone other than the nurse or met by the patient themselves, they may have been overlooked.

Table 4.7 illustrates that nurses perceived spiritual need in a variety of ways. Three points can be noted from this table, each of which is discussed in turn.

First, the fact that the highest proportion of nurses (34.2%) viewed spiritual need as the need for belief and faith, 31.3% considering it to be religious in nature, suggests that nurses seemed to view spiritual need in religious terms. This implies that patients' religious needs may have been better recognised than other spiritual needs e.g., for hope and creativity.

The literature review highlighted that all people have spiritual needs, regardless of the possession of religious beliefs. Nurses who viewed spiritual need in religious terms only, therefore, may fail to identify spiritual needs in patients who claim no religious affiliation or may assume certain spiritual needs in those claiming a particular religious affiliation. In both cases, patients' true spiritual needs may not be recognised. Alternatively, given that the study targeted nurses who were caring for the elderly, and that the elderly may have tended to express their spirituality through religion, it may have been that the spiritual needs patients experienced were predominantly religious.

Second, the literature consistently considered the needs for MPF and hope as spiritual needs. The study findings, however, do not appear to be in keeping with the literature as only 9.9% and 3.6% of nurses respectively defined spiritual need in these ways. This implies that nurses may not have addressed the fundamental spiritual needs of MPF and hope or it may have been that the elderly found meaning and hope through religious experiences and practices. Alternatively, nurses may have considered the needs for MPF and hope/creativity as psychological rather than spiritual in nature. This is possible given that 1.5% nurses in the miscellaneous category viewed spiritual need in this way. If nurses viewed the needs for MPF and hope as psychological rather than spiritual in nature the danger is that these needs could have been inadequately catered for because spiritual interventions were ignored.

Third, in the miscellaneous category (Table 4.7), 3.9% of nurses expressed difficulty in defining spiritual need. This small percentage could be representative of the non-respondent group, e.g., two of the 22 nurses who chose not to complete the questionnaire did so because they found the questions difficult to answer (Table 4.16). Thus it could be that the proportion of nurses in the population who were unclear about what spiritual needs were and therefore unsure about what spiritual care involved, was higher than the study findings indicated.

The indicators nurses used in identifying patients' spiritual needs are outlined in Table 4.11. Given that the common theme in indicators 2-6 and part of indicator 1 is non-verbal/indirect verbal communication, it would seem, therefore, that nurses were mainly alerted to patients' spiritual needs in this way. This finding suggests that spiritual needs may be more subtle and more difficult to identify than other needs e.g., certain physical needs.

Planning and intervention Almost all nurses (93.7%) (Table 4.9) considered it their shared responsibility, with the clergy (73.5%) and others (20.2%) to respond to patients' spiritual needs. The fact that over half (51.6%) in Table 4.8 referred these needs suggests, however, that most nurses either felt unable to respond or did not consider it their duty to personally respond to patients' spiritual needs. Whatever the reasons, the fact that over half of nurses felt personally unable to respond, referral being the preferred option, suggests that spiritual care may lack continuity.

Some nurses (Table 4.8) such as those who were prepared to 'be with' the patient (18.8%) or listen to/talk with the patient about their situation (6.5%), were however willing to respond personally to patients' spiritual needs. Why some nurses felt personally able to respond whilst others did not was not clear. Additionally, it was not known which spiritual needs the former group of nurses felt able to respond personally.

It is noteworthy that, although 31.3% of nurses viewed spiritual need in religious terms (Table 4.7), only 6.7% considered spiritual care to involve facilitating participation in religious rituals (Table 4.8). This could be explained if nurses referred patients' religious needs to others.

Evaluation As illustrated in Table 4.12, the majority of nurses (84.4%) considered the interventions employed to meet patients' spiritual needs to have been either totally (29.2%) or partially (55.2%) effective. A minority (4.6%), however, were of the opinion that the care given had been ineffective to a greater or lesser degree.

As Table 4.13 shows, nurses evaluated the effectiveness of the spiritual care given mainly through observing non-verbal/indirect verbal cues given by patients which were the opposite of those alerting them to patients' spiritual needs in the first place.

It would seem that all but 11% of nurses (Table 4.12) were able to evaluate the spiritual care given. As the majority would or did refer spiritual needs to others (51.6%, Table 4.8), this would suggest that nurses did not have to be personally involved in responding to patients' spiritual needs to be able to evaluate the extent to which their needs had been met.

Probably because the majority of nurses considered the spiritual care given to have been effective, only 10.1% stated they would have responded differently to patients' spiritual needs (Table 4.14). Over half of these nurses (51.1%) would have referred to others (Table 4.15) which may highlight these nurses feelings of inadequacy in dealing with patients' spiritual concerns. Other nurses (26.7%, Table 4.15) would have liked to have spent more time with patients/family which suggests that lack of time could interfere with the practice of spiritual care.

Additionally some nurses found it difficult to evaluate the spiritual care given (11%. Table 4.12) mainly because of patients' unresponsiveness (9.7%, Table 4.13) which highlights Hockey's (1979) finding that patient characteristics can influence the nursing care given (Figure 2.2).

Reasons for nurses not completing the questionnaire A very small percentage (3.2%) of nurses stated their reasons for choosing not to complete the questionnaire. As previously mentioned, it was thought that the reasons nurses gave for not completing the questionnaire (Table 4.16) might highlight possible characteristics of the non-respondent group (32.2% of the population). As Table 4.16 shows, a wide variety of reasons were given by nurses. The majority (17 out of 22, or 77%), however, did not complete the questionnaire because they either did not consider spiritual care part of their role (seven out of 22 nurses, reasons 1 and 3) or felt unable to give it (10 out of 22 nurses, reasons 2, 6 and 7).

Discussion of results in relation to the literature In the following discussion, the study findings are compared with the literature. As in the previous section, the discussion follows the stages of the nursing process.

As outlined in Part 1, comparisons between studies were made difficult by the fact that operational definitions of terms were frequently lacking or were not cited in summarised versions of the original studies. There was no guarantee, therefore, that the terminology used was consistent across studies. In addition each study had its own limitations.

Assessment Whereas in this study the majority (76.8%) of nurses said they had identified a spiritual need at some point in their practice, there was conflicting evidence of this in the other available research.

In Chadwick's (1975) study all nurses stated they had recognised a spiritual need at some time as did the majority in Chance's (1967) study. Additionally Piles (1986) highlighted how 30.7%-50.6% of nurses 'often' assessed more general aspects of the patient's spiritual state but that only 15.8%-18.7% 'often' assessed more specific aspects of patients' spiritual needs and 61% 'seldom/never' diagnosed spiritual distress.

Other studies highlighted that nurses had a limited awareness of patients' spiritual needs (Highfield and Cason, 1983). Only 29.5% of nurses in Kramer's

(1957) study considered it their duty to identify a spiritual need for referral to the clergy. Furthermore O'Neill (1984) found that patients' religious needs were not recorded in nursing records.

Collectively as a group nurses' definitions of spiritual need in this study covered all aspects of the operational definition derived from the literature. In addition, nurses mentioned two other aspects of spiritual need not covered by the operational definition. The first was the need for peace and comfort which was more in keeping with indicators of spiritual well-being cited by Highfield and Cason (1983). The second concerned aspects of the miscellaneous category where 4.7% and 3.1% of nurses respectively defined spiritual need in terms of an individual need and deeper need than any other. These definitions were more akin to the descriptions of the spiritual dimension presented in Part 1.

The finding that nurses tended to equate spiritual needs with religious needs was similar to other studies (Chance, 1967; Highfield and Cason, 1983; Piles, 1986; Samarel, 1991).

Patients in most other studies reported having experienced spiritual needs which included the need for: meaning; belief in God, often expressed through formal religious practices; relatedness to others/God; relief from conditions such as fear, doubt, loneliness (Martin et al., 1976; Simsen, 1985; Stallwood-Hess, 1969). The fact that all these needs expressed by patients were similarly considered to be spiritual in nature by nurses in this study suggests nurses may be in a good position to be able to identify and respond to these needs.

Chance's (1967) finding was similar to this study in that nurses were mainly alerted to patients' spiritual needs through non-verbal/indirect verbal means of communication, e.g., emotional attitudes, tears, gestures. Additionally many of the indicators of spiritual distress and well-being could be considered to be non-verbal.

Planning and intervention Nurses, both in this and other studies seemed to prefer to refer patients' spiritual needs to others rather than responding to them personally (Chance, 1967; Kealey, 1974; Piles, 1986). Patients in other studies similarly considered the clergy and nurse to have a major role in spiritual care followed by others such as family and friends (Table 4.17). It was suggested by the author and highlighted by other studies (Chadwick, 1973; Highfield and Cason, 1983; Kealey, 1974; Kramer, 1957; Piles, 1986) that nurses may have referred patients' spiritual needs because they felt inadequate about giving spiritual care.

Referral of spiritual needs is all very well provided that clergy, etc. are available. Only one study (Byles, 1961) was identified which addressed hospitals' provision of clergy and in this instance only children's' hospitals in parts of the USA were selected. In over 50% of these hospitals (n=133)

Table 4.17
Sources of help in spiritual care mentioned by patients in other studies

Rank	Person patients considered could help them with their spiritual needs	Author(s) of study
1	Clergy	Martin et al., 1976
	Clergy	Stallwood-Hess, 1969
	Anyone else (excluding clergy, nurses and any other members of the HCT).	Chomicz ,1984
	Met alone	Kealey, 1974
2	Nurses.	Chomicz, 1984
	Nurses	Stallwood-Hess, 1969
	God	Kealey, 1974
	Family	Martin et al., 1976
3	Family	Stallwood-Hess, 1969
	Family, friends and clergy	Kealey, 1974
	Clergy	Chomicz, 1984
	Nurse	Martin et al., 1976
4	Friends	Martin et al., 1976
	Friends	Stallwood-Hess, 1969
	Other hospital staff (other than nurse, clergy)	Chomicz ,1984
5	Doctor	Martin et al., 1976
	Psychiatrist	Stallwood-Hess, 1969
6	Other hospital staff (other than clergy, nurses, psychiatrist)	Stallwood-Hess, 1969
	God	Martin et al., 1976

Source: Author's own

policies stated that nurses should refer spiritual matters to others, especially the chaplain, yet less than 20% of hospitals had a full time chaplain and over

50% had no available official chaplain. Thus, although referral appeared to be an accepted intervention, the resources may not have been adequate. Further research would be required to ascertain British hospitals' provision of clergy.

Although over half of the nurses in this study preferred to give spiritual care by referring, it was noted that some (18.8%) would do so by 'being with' the patient. This concept of nurses giving spiritual care by their presence and by the use of touch was also noted in other studies (Piles, 1986, Martin, et al., 1976, Samarel, 1991, Stallwood-Hess, 1969).

Furthermore, some (6.7%) nurses considered spiritual care to involve facilitating participation in religious rituals. In other British studies there was conflicting evidence as to whether or not patients considered religious practices important to them (Chomicz, 1984, Simsen, 1985). Of those patients who did (Chomicz, 1984), the acts of taking communion and attending church services were cited as the most important. Generally American nurses stated that they would feel comfortable about helping patients with prayer and in the reading of religious literature (Chadwick, 1973, Chance, 1967, Kealey, 1974, Kramer, 1957), however two studies indicated that, in practice, they tended not to do so (Chadwick, 1973, Piles ,1986).

There would appear to be some discrepancy, therefore, between nurses' intentions and actions. There could be a number of reasons for this. It may be that the majority of patients do not consider religious practices important to them, as was found by Chomicz (1984) or it may be that they do (Simsen, 1985) but do not consider the nurse the most appropriate person to help in this way. For example the majority of patients (58%) in one study (Martin et al., 1976) said they would not like the nurse to pray with/read scripture to them and in another (Kealey 1974) the majority met their spiritual needs through communicating with God personally. Alternatively other factors such as lack of time, as highlighted earlier in this section, may have prevented nurses from carrying out their intentions.

Another group of nurses (6.5%) in this study considered that spiritual care could be given through listening to and talking with patients. Nurses and patients in other studies were also of this opinion (Chance, 1967, Kealey, 1974, Piles, 1986, Stallwood-Hess, 1969) and in one study (Martin et al., 1976) the majority (77%) of patients considered that nurses could help most by listening.

Evaluation The majority of nurses in this study (84.4%) considered the spiritual care given to have been effective. This was a similar finding to that of Chadwick (1973), the only other study identified which addressed nurses' evaluations of spiritual care.

One would expect that if effective spiritual care had been given then patients' would have expressed satisfaction with the care they had received. Other studies indicated that in general patients' felt their spiritual needs had been met to some extent (Martin et al., 1976, Stallwood-Hess, 1969). No studies were identified, however, which examined both nurses' and patients' perspectives, therefore, further research which addresses both these issues would be required to ascertain the efficacy of the spiritual care given.

Summary

Although there was conflicting evidence in other studies, within the sample in this study, the majority of nurses claimed to have identified a spiritual need in a patient at some point in their practice. It was not possible, however, to determine the extent to which they had done so.

Collectively as a group nurses' perceptions of spiritual need covered all aspects of the operational definition derived from the literature. They viewed it in terms of the individual's need for belief and faith; for peace and comfort; to give and receive love and forgiveness; for MPF; for hope and creativity. They tended, however, to view spiritual need more in religious terms which could indicate that patients' religious needs might be better identified than other spiritual needs. Furthermore, nurses were alerted to patients' spiritual needs mainly through recognising non-verbal/indirect verbal cues patients displayed.

Although the majority of nurses considered it their shared responsibility to respond to patients' spiritual needs and some were prepared to be personally involved in this, the majority seemed to prefer to refer these needs to others possibly because they felt inadequate. This finding was similarly reflected in other studies.

Nurses seemed able to evaluate the effectiveness of the spiritual care patients' had received even if they had not been personally involved in giving this care. Their evaluations were mainly positive and they reached their decision predominantly through observing non-verbal/indirect verbal cues given by patients.

There is suggestion that, as illustrated by Hockey (1979) (Figure 2.2), nurse, patient and environment related factors may have influenced the spiritual care patients received.

Moreover, lack of time and aspects of the patient's condition e.g., if confused or unresponsive, seemed to hinder some nurses from giving spiritual care.

Having described how nurses perceived spiritual need and spiritual care and how they reported to have given this care attention focuses in the following section, on identifying factors which appeared to influence the spiritual care given.

Factors which appeared to influence the spiritual care given

Factors were identified by exploring nurses' responses in the questionnaire and by cross-tabulating certain variables in SPSS. Each approach is explained in turn before the findings are summarised.

Exploration of nurses' responses

A number of factors emerged from the responses nurses gave in the questionnaire which appeared to influence their giving of spiritual care. These factors were similar to those identified by Hockey (1979) (Figure 2.2) and were related to the nurse, patient and environment. Each is discussed in turn.

Concerning the nurse, it was suggested by the author that, as patients' spiritual needs were mainly recognised through non-verbal/indirect verbal cues given by the patient, these needs may be more difficult to identify than other needs. Whether or not spiritual needs were recognised may, therefore, be dependent on the sensitivity of the individual nurse. For instance, a nurse who is insensitive may not pick up on the non-verbal/indirect verbal cues given by the patient, therefore, the patient's spiritual needs could remain unrecognised.

Furthermore, it seemed that some nurses personally responded to patients' spiritual needs whereas others did not. The way in which nurses responded may have been related to their perception of spiritual need and spiritual care and their perception of their role in and ability to give this care, as explained below.

It was suggested that the proportion of nurses in the population who were unclear of what spiritual needs were and therefore unsure of what spiritual care involved, may have been higher than indicated by the study findings. For a substantial proportion of the population, their uncertainty with regard to what spiritual needs and spiritual care were may have prevented them from identifying or personally responding to patients' spiritual needs.

The findings revealed that over half of nurses felt personally unable to respond to patients' spiritual needs. The fact that seven out of 22 nurses indicated that they did not complete the questionnaire because they did not consider spiritual care to be part of their role (Table 4.16) suggests that, whether or not patients' spiritual needs are identified and the way in which nurses respond to these needs, may depend on their perception of their role in spiritual care.

There is a possible alternative explanation. As discussed above, over half of the nurses referred patients' spiritual needs. Furthermore, over half (51.1%) of those who stated they would have responded differently would also have referred (Table 4.15) and ten out of 22 nurses did not complete the questionnaire because they felt unable to give spiritual care (Table 4.16). Thus it would appear that some nurses may not have responded personally to patients' spiritual needs because they perceived themselves to be inadequate. If the nurses who had opted not to complete the questionnaire were representative of the non-respondent group (n=377, Table 4.5) this would mean that 290 (77% of 377) nurses may have failed to identify spiritual needs and/or give spiritual care because they either did not consider it their duty or felt unable to. Thus the proportion of nurses not identifying patients' spiritual needs and, therefore, not giving spiritual care may have been higher than the findings indicate. Patients' spiritual needs may, therefore, have been less well catered for than the study findings suggest.

In addition to nurse related factors, those connected with the patient also appeared to influence the spiritual care nurses gave. One nurse had not completed the questionnaire because she was unable to identify spiritual needs in the confused elderly for whom she was looking after (Table 4.16) whilst others reported difficulty in evaluating the spiritual care given to patients who were unresponsive (Table 4.13). Thus factors in the patient's condition which interfered with nurse-patient communication seemed to make it difficult for some nurses to give spiritual care and further highlights Hockey's (1979) finding (Figure 2.2) that characteristics of the patient may influence the care nurses give.

Concerning environmental factors, lack of time seemed to interfere with the giving of spiritual care (Table 4.15).

In summary, having explored nurses responses in the questionnaire it would seem that nurse, patient and environment related factors appeared to influence the spiritual care some nurses gave.

Cross-tabulation of variables using SPSS

In order to identify, more reliably, factors which may have influenced the spiritual care nurses gave, variables were cross-tabulated using SPSS. Only factors found to be significant at the 95% level are reported. Four factors, namely geographical location, ward type and the grade and belief system of the nurse were found to be significantly associated with the identification of spiritual needs by nurses. The results are presented in a series of tables before they are discussed.

Presentation of results

Health Board area As table 4.18 shows, there were variations between Health Boards in the percentage of nurses who had identified spiritual needs.

Table 4.18
Proportion of respondents in each Health Board who had identified a spiritual need

Health Board	No	%
Argyll & Clyde	53	91.4
Western Isles	13	86.7
Greater Glasgow	103	83.1
Lothian	102	82.9
Highland	21	80.8
Lanarkshire	26	76.5
Shetland	3	75.0
Grampian	72	72.0
Tayside	50	69.4
Forth Valley	29	67.4
Borders	7	63.6
Dumfries & Galloway	24	53.3

Source: Author's own

Ward type   Ward types were classified into two groups as follows.

1   Nurses working in non-varied wards, i.e., chronic geriatric ward only or acute geriatric ward only. Included were:

'long term care' only

'geriatric assessment' and/or 'geriatric medicine' only.

2   Nurses working on varied wards i.e., acute and chronic care combined. Included were:

'acute and chronic geriatric wards combined'

'chronic geriatric wards combined with other wards outwith care of the elderly'

'acute geriatric wards combined with other wards outwith care of the elderly' 'acute and chronic geriatric wards combined with other wards outwith care of the elderly'.

The results are shown in Table 4.19 below.

Table 4.19
Proportion of respondents in each ward type who had identified a spiritual need

Ward type	Had identified a spiritual need	
	No.	%
Non-varied	307	73.1
Varied	196	83.4

Source: Author's own

As Table 4.19 shows, a higher proportion of nurses working on varied wards claimed to have identified spiritual needs compared with those working on non-varied wards.

Grade of the nurse

As shown in Table 4.20, a higher proportion of C/N's than S/N's had identified a spiritual need.

Table 4.20
Proportion of C/N's and S/N's who had identified a spiritual need

Grade	Had identified a spiritual need	
	No.	%
C/N	216	81.6
S/N	240	72.1

Source: Author's own

128

Table 4.21
According to their profession of religious affiliation, proportion of respondents who had identified a spiritual need

Profession of religious affiliation	Had identified a spiritual need	
	No.	%
Yes	340	79.4
No	154	72.0

Source: Author's own

Belief system of the nurse

As Table 4.21 illustrates, a higher proportion of nurses professing religious affiliation had identified a spiritual need than those claiming none. In order to determine if nurses with particular types of religious affiliation identified spiritual needs more readily than others, the two variables were cross-tabulated. Because there were too many groups with low numbers to enable conclusions to be drawn, the fifteen types of religious affiliation were merged into five groups namely:

1　Roman Catholic.

2　Anglican/Episcopalian.

3　Non-Anglican Protestant.

4　Combination of all other formal religious groups (Pentecostal, Baptist/ Brethren, Methodist, Salvation Army, Quakers, Free Church, Moslem, two or more categories).

5　Other (cults/occult, those who believed in something, did not wish to reveal type of religious affiliation, atheist/humanists).

The results are presented in Table 4.22 on p.130.

Nurses with beliefs not obviously connected with religion ('other' group) were most likely to have identified a spiritual need, closely followed jointly by those in the Roman Catholic and combined religious groups.

Nurses who claimed to be Anglican or non-Anglican Protestants were less likely to have identified spiritual needs.

Table 4.22
Proportion of respondents claiming a particular type of religious affiliation, who had identified a spiritual need

Type of religious affiliation	Had identified a spiritual need	
	No.	%
Roman Catholics.	84	88.4
Anglicans/Episcopalians.	17	70.8
Non-Anglican protestant.	163	74.8
All other formal religious groups combined.	38	88.4
Other	24	88.9

Source: Author's own

In summary, having cross-tabulated variables using SPSS the geographical location of the nurse, the type of ward in which she was working, together with her grade and belief system were factors which appeared to be associated with the identification of spiritual needs by nurses. Each finding is discussed in turn below and possible explanations are explored.

Discussion of results

Geographical location No explanation could be identified for the finding that higher percentages of nurses in certain Health Boards identified spiritual needs. It was thought that nurses in these Health Boards may have defined spiritual need in broader terms and, therefore, may have classified a broader range of needs as spiritual compared with nurses who viewed the concept more narrowly. Cross-tabulation of the relevant variables, however, revealed no such association.

Alternatively it was thought that the finding may have been attributable to a factor other than the geographical location of respondents. For instance it could have been that higher proportions of C/N's were located in Health Boards where the highest proportions of nurses reported having identified spiritual needs. This, however, was not the case.

Ward type Although a number of reasons are suggested, exactly why a higher percentage of nurses working on varied wards should have reported identifying patients' spiritual needs compared with those working on non-varied wards was not clear.

There is suggestion from Reed and Bond's (1991) work that nurses working on long term care of the elderly wards (non-varied) may experience little satisfaction in their work if they aim for the inappropriate and unachievable goals of cure and/or rehabilitation. It was thought, therefore, that nurses working on varied wards may have experienced greater job satisfaction than those working on non-varied wards which may be more conducive to them maintaining a questioning attitude. They may, therefore, have been more alert to patients' needs in general and, therefore, to their spiritual needs in particular.

Alternatively, unresponsiveness of patients was a factor identified in the previous section which appeared to hinder nurses from giving spiritual care. It is possible that patients in non-varied wards were less responsive than those in varied wards thereby making it more difficult for nurses to identify their spiritual needs.

Moreover, given that there could have been a higher proportion of physically dependent patients located in non-varied wards, this could have meant that nurses on these wards had less time to devote to spiritual care.

Grade It was not clear why more C/N's than S/N's claimed to have identified patients' spiritual needs.

It was thought that the identification of spiritual needs may have been a skill acquired with age and experience and that as C/N's were probably older and more experienced than S/N's, this could have explained why they were more likely to have identified spiritual needs. However, although C/N's were significantly older and had been significantly longer in practice than S/N's, no associations were found between age or the length of time in practice and the identification of spiritual needs. The maturity and ability of the nurse to learn may have been more important than her age and length of time in practice in determining her ability to identify patients' spiritual needs. It could have been that these were qualities C/N's possessed in greater measure than S/N's.

Alternatively, it was considered that C/N's may have identified spiritual needs if they were more religious or perhaps perceived spiritual need and spiritual care differently from S/N's. No such associations were, however, found.

Finally, it was suggested that certain aspects of the C/N's role may have given them a certain advantage over S/N's in identifying patients' spiritual needs.

As the key person the C/N may have been privy to more information about patients from a greater number of sources than the S/N and, being less directly involved in giving patient care, she may have been more able to adopt an objective view of the 'total' patient. These factors, combined with her overall responsibility for the total well-being of patients under her care and possibly greater opportunity to attend courses and study days, may have put the C/N in a better position to identify patients' spiritual needs than the S/N. These suggestions are, however, merely speculative and further research would be required to explore the issue of role differences in relation to the identification of spiritual needs.

Belief system It was not clear why a higher percentage of nurses who claimed religious affiliation identified spiritual needs than those claiming none.

There was no difference in the way either of the groups perceived spiritual need or spiritual care. Furthermore, although those who professed to having a religious affiliation were significantly older than those who did not, it cannot be assumed that they were more likely to identify spiritual needs because they were more mature. Further research would be required to ascertain this.

No explanation could be found either to explain why higher percentages of nurses claiming certain types of religious affiliation identified spiritual need than others. Again there was no difference between the groups in terms of their perceptions of spiritual needs and spiritual care. It was thought that conservatism of belief might offer an explanation, however the only group found to be conservative in their belief was the combined religious group. Conservatism of belief could not, therefore, explain why higher percentages of Roman Catholic nurses and those who held beliefs not obviously connected with religion had identified patients' spiritual needs than those in the other groups.

In summary, although no explanations could be found, C/N's claiming religious affiliation and working on varied wards in certain geographical locations seemed most likely to have identified patients' spiritual needs.

14 Summary

In this section attention has focused on the first stage of the of the study, namely the quantitative approach.

The way in which nurses, within the sample, perceived spiritual need and spiritual care and gave this care in practice was described. It was also found that certain factors, similar to those identified by Hockey (1979) (Figure 2.2), appeared to influence the spiritual care nurses gave. These factors were related to the nurse, the environment in which she was working and the patients for whom she was caring and are summarised in Figure 4.15.

In order to further explore the factors which appeared to influence the spiritual care nurses gave, a different approach was adopted and is described in Part 5.

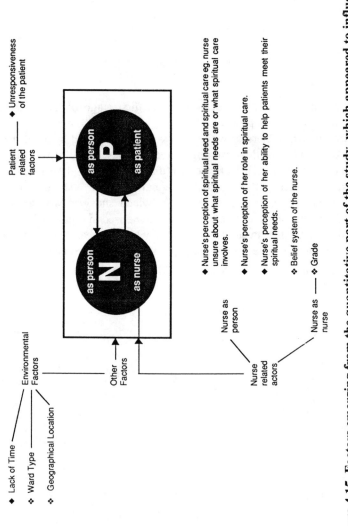

Figure 4.15 Factors emerging from the quantitative part of the study, which appeared to influence spiritual care

Source: Author's own

134

Part Five
QUALITATIVE APPROACH

15 Aim and method

This section describes the second part of the study, namely the qualitative approach. The aim and method are outlined before the results are presented, discussed and conclusions drawn.

As discussed in Part 4, several factors emerged from the quantitative part of the study which appeared to influence the spiritual care nurses gave. It was in an attempt to further explore these factors that semi-structured interviews were conducted with a sample of nurses. Although it was acknowledged that, because of the sample size, the results would not be generalisable, it was considered that they would make a valuable contribution in highlighting possible factors which may have influenced the spiritual care given by the sample of nurses.

Design of the interview schedule

As the purpose of the interviews was to explore individual nurses' experiences in greater depth than had been achieved through the questionnaire, both standard questions and those relevant to the individual nurse's experiences were included in the interview schedule.

Selection of the sample

It emerged from analysis of data in the quantitative part of the study that there was a geographical difference in the identification of spiritual needs by nurses (Part 4). The sample of nurses for interview was, therefore, selected from three Health Boards namely: Argyll and Clyde which had the highest percentage of nurses identifying spiritual needs; Dumfries and Galloway which had the lowest percentage; Lothian which was in the middle range and was also practical in terms of travel.

Nurses were divided into four groups as follows:

1 Those who stated they had not identified a spiritual need.

2 Those who stated they had identified a spiritual need but did not say how they had recognised it, responded or evaluated the care given.

3 Those who stated they had identified a spiritual need and considered their interventions to have been totally effective.

4 Those who stated they had identified a spiritual need but considered their interventions to have been more ineffective than effective.

Because of the time constraints it was not possible to interview all nurses in all four groups. It was intended, therefore, to select, from each Health Board, one nurse from each of the four groups for interview, i..e., twelve nurses. However, as only one nurse met with the criteria for Group 2, this left ten potential interviewees who were selected on the basis of the following criteria.

Their belief system

As nurses' profession of religious affiliation had emerged as a significant factor in the identification of patients' spiritual needs (Part 4) it was considered important to include nurses with and without religious affiliation.

Their stated responses

Some nurses responded personally to patients' spiritual needs whereas others did not (Table 4.8). By including both types of nurses it was hoped to isolate factors which may have influenced the way in which they responded.

Their stated evaluations

Some nurses appeared to evaluate the effectiveness of care given by focusing on the patient e.g., patient seemed content, whereas others did so on the basis of whether or not an event had occurred, e.g., the minister had visited (Table 4.13). By targeting both types of nurses it was intended to elicit factors which appeared to determine how they evaluated spiritual care.

Where there were several nurses to choose from in relation to the above criteria, those who gave the most comprehensive answers were selected.

Researcher bias was acknowledged in this process. Where there was no obvious difference between responses, nurses were chosen at random.

In this way ten nurses were selected for interview. On checking the sample these nurses represented all grades and ward types, factors which were previously identified in association with the recognition of spiritual needs by nurses (Part 4).

As all nurses in the sample who had identified a spiritual need also claimed some form of religious affiliation, it was decided to add a nurse, from Lothian Health Board for ease of travel, who had identified a spiritual need but claimed no religious affiliation.

Out of interest it was decided also to include an atheist in the sample, although it was acknowledged that this provided no basis for any assumption about atheism in nursing. Two atheists were identified, one in Tayside Health Board and another in Grampian. As the latter had left employment the former was included.

The final sample, therefore, consisted of 12 nurses who varied in their geographical location, grade, ward type, belief system and the way in which they responded to patients' spiritual needs and evaluated the care given.

Operationalisation of the qualitative part of the study

Having selected the sample, the appropriate hospitals were telephoned to check that the nurses were still working there. Forwarding addresses of those who had changed employment were obtained. All twelve nurses were then invited to participate in semi-structured tape recorded interviews at venues of their choice. They were asked to complete and return a form detailing their home telephone number and the most convenient time for the researcher to telephone to arrange a time for interview. Consent was assumed when nurses gave this information. Where replies had not been received ten days after the mailing of the first letter, a reminder letter was sent. In instances where this failed to achieve a response a substitute nurse was contacted using the procedure already described.

All interviews were conducted by the researcher who was aware of the bias that this would introduce. In eleven of the interviews the researcher met with the nurses and tape recorded the sessions. A telephone interview took place with the nurse from Tayside Health Board because the travelling which would have been required to conduct one interview was considered uneconomical.

All interviews were transcribed.

Analysis of the interviews

It appeared to the researcher that different nurses identified different types of spiritual needs and that they recognised them, responded and evaluated at different levels as illustrated in Figure 5.1. Thus, overall, some nurses gave spiritual care at a deeper level than others as shown in Figure 5.2.

The spiritual needs nurses identified and the care they reported to have given were, therefore, classified according to the types of need and levels of care illustrated in Figure 5.1.

Factors which appeared to influence the spiritual care nurses gave were elicited by examining the interview transcripts namely by:

1 Noting nurses' explanations for some of the findings in the quantitative part of the study.

2 Identifying factors nurses' suggested did/could influence the spiritual care given.

3 Exploring with nurses some of their responses in the questionnaire.

4 Noting factors which, according to the researcher, appeared to have some bearing on the spiritual care nurses gave.

5 Exploring characteristics of nurses in relation to the level of spiritual care they gave.

The results of each of the above analyses are presented in turn in the following section.

Although the researcher endeavoured to conduct the above analyses as objectively as possible, researcher bias could not be ruled out. The reader is reminded that references to what nurses 'did' refers to what they 'said they did'.

SPIRITUAL NEEDS

TYPE 1   TYPE 2

➤ TYPE 1

Needs which are obviously religious

➤ TYPE 2

Needs not obviously connected with religion

RECOGNITION OF NEEDS

1st level
2nd level

➤ 1st Level

Need communicated more obviously. Includes:
- need voiced directly by patient
- need noted because of patient's religious behaviour e.g. reading Bible, praying aloud
- need noted because of avoidance behaviour of the patient in relation to religious activities
- need suspected because of patient's religious affiliation
- need assumed because of fact that patient is human, patient's situation

➤ 2nd Level

Need is perceived at a deeper level i.e. through:
- knowing patient
- sharing of self
- sensing
- observation and interpretation of comments/behaviour not obviously connected with religion

RESPONSE TO NEEDS

1st level
2nd level
3rd level

➤ 1st Level

Minimal personal nurse involvement e.g:
- reffering to someone else
- allowing access of religious groups
- arranging for rituals to be performed

➤ 2nd Level

Some personal nurse involvement but not on a deep personal level e.g:
- listening
- giving good care
- talking on a superficial level e.g. about day's events

➤ 3rd Level

Active personal involvement on a deep level e.g:
- empathy
- "being with" patient
- actively exploring situation with patient
- sharing of self

EVALUATION OF RESPONSE

1st level
2nd level
3rd level

➤ 1st Level

Didn't know or found it difficult to evaluate

➤ 2nd Level

Evaluation on basis of:
- fact that an act was completed
- verbal comments from patient
- behaviour of patient in response to some action having been taken

➤ 3rd Level

Evaluation involving perception at a deeper level e.g:
- sensing
- observation and interpretation of non-verbal/more subtle cues

Figure 5.1 Types of spiritual needs identified by nurses and the level of spiritual care given

Source: Author's own

141

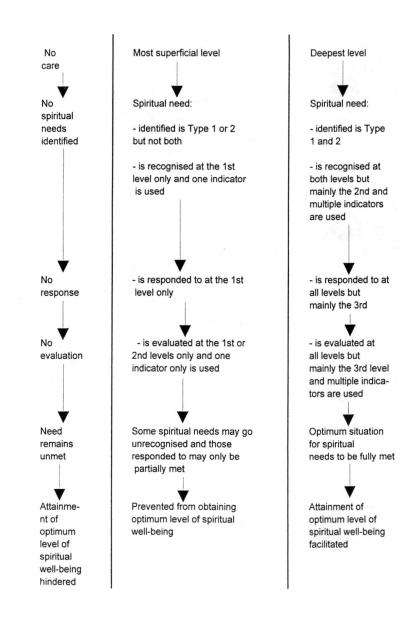

Figure 5.2 Levels at which spiritual care, as an entity, can be given
Source: Author's own

16 Results

Nurses' explanations for some of the findings

Interviewees were asked if they could think of possible reasons for the associations found between grade and ward type, and the identification of spiritual needs by nurses. Of the 12 nurses interviewed, eight offered explanations.

Nurses considered that C/N's may have been in a better position to identify patients' spiritual needs than S/N's because of their overall responsibility for patient care, together with the fact that they are usually privy to more information and less involved in giving nursing care. Similar suggestions had previously been given by the author (Part 4, Section 12).

Also, in a similar vein to the author (Part 4, Section 12), they felt that nurses working on non-varied wards may have reported identifying fewer spiritual needs than those working on varied wards because staff may have been more institutionalised or patients less communicative. In addition they suggested that nurses working on varied wards may have had greater exposure to acute situations involving unexpected or untimely death than nurses working on non-varied wards where death may have been an expected outcome. Nurses may, therefore, have been more likely to encounter the 'why' questions and those concerned with meaning which are fundamental spiritual issues.

Factors nurses suggested did/could influence the spiritual care given

In the course of the interviews nurses suggested a number of factors which they felt had or could have influenced the spiritual care given to patients. These factors are illustrated in Figure 5.3 and are clustered under the headings used by Hockey (1979) (Figure 2.2). In brackets beside each factor, the number of nurses who were of this opinion is stated.

Figure 5.3 shows that nurses considered a wide variety of factors as influential in spiritual care. These included factors relating to the nurse, the support of other professionals, the environment in which she was working, and the type of patients for whom she was caring.

Exploration with nurses of some of their responses in the questionnaire

In the questionnaire some nurses stated that they had not identified any spiritual needs. Others stated they had but did not indicate if or how they had responded whilst others evaluated the care given from totally effective to more ineffective than effective. By exploring at interview their written responses, it was hoped to obtain some idea of the factors which appeared to prevent nurses from identifying and responding to patients' spiritual needs and those which hindered or facilitated effective spiritual care from being given. Each is discussed in turn.

Factors which appeared to prevent nurses from identifying spiritual needs

Three nurses in the sample stated that they had not identified spiritual needs, the reasons given by them being connected with their belief system.

First they equated spiritual needs with religious needs. As they did not consider themselves to be religious people or to know much about the subject, they felt unable to identify these needs in patients. They indicated that education with regard to the latter would be of no benefit to them because they did not consider spiritual care to be part of the nurse's role.

Second, as they were of the opinion that peoples' beliefs were a personal and private matter, they considered it inappropriate for them to ask patients about their spiritual needs.

It emerged at interview that all three nurses who had originally stated that they had not identified any spiritual needs had actually done so, but they had only become aware of this through discussion.

The spiritual needs recognised by them were exclusively concerned with patients' religious needs, e.g., to attend mass, and were identified at the most superficial level, e.g., through patients' voicing their needs directly. Furthermore, nurses responded to these needs with the minimum of personal involvement e.g., contacted the priest, and evaluated the care given by the fact that an act had been completed, e.g., the priest had visited.

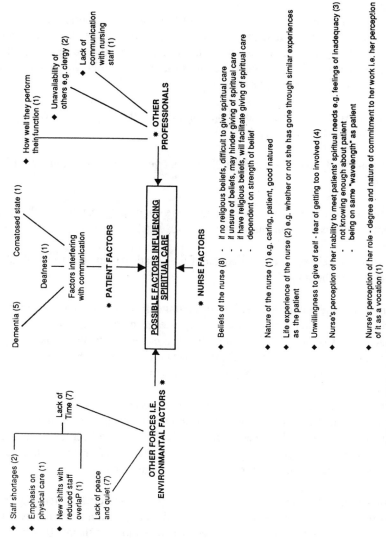

Staff shortages (2)

◆ Emphasis on physical care (1)

◆ New shifts with reduced staff overlaP (1)

Lack of Time (7)

Lack of peace and quiet (7)

OTHER FORCES I.E. ENVIRONMANTAL FACTORS *

Dementia (5)   Comatosed state (1)

Deafness (1)

Factors interfering with communication

* PATIENT FACTORS

◆ How well they perform thein function (1)

◆ Unavailability of others e.g. clergy (2)

◆ Lack of communication with nursing staff (1)

* OTHER PROFESSIONALS

┌─────────────────────┐
│ **POSSIBLE FACTORS INFLUENCING** │
│ **SPIRITUAL CARE** │
└─────────────────────┘

* NURSE FACTORS

◆ Beliefs of the nurse (8) -   if no religious beliefs, difficult to give spiritual care
        - if unsure of beliefs, may hinder giving of spiritual care
        - if have religious beliefs, will facilitate giving of spiritual care
        - dependent on strength of belief

◆ Nature of the nurse (1) e.g. caring, patient, good natured

◆ Life experience of the nurse (2) e.g. whether or not she has gone through similar experiences as the patient

◆ Unwillingness to give of self - fear of getting too involved (4)

◆ Nurse's perception of her inability to meet patients' spiritual needs e.g. feelings of inadequacy (3)
        - not knowing enough about patient
        - being on same "wavelength" as patient

◆ Nurse's perception of her role - degree and nature of commitment to her work i.e. her perception of it as a vocation (1)

Figure 5.3 Factors nurses suggested could/did influence the spiritual care given

Source: Author's own

145

These nurses also demonstrated a number of other characteristics as described below.

1 They did not seem to know much about the spiritual dimension in general. For instance, they stated they were lacking in knowledge in this respect, had never really thought about it before and found the questions in the questionnaire difficult to answer as illustrated by the following quotations taken from their transcripts:

...you were making me think about all sorts of things that I don't usually delve into in any great depth.

...I don't really like this question...I find that very difficult (defining spiritual need).

2 They perceived themselves as inadequate in helping patients with their spiritual needs e.g., one nurse said openly:

...I would feel extremely inadequate if they (patient) did start to speak like that to me (about God)...

Another nurse stated that the lack of courage of the nurse might be a factor which would determine whether or not she gave spiritual care. She said that she was personally afraid of getting too close to patients. This perhaps reflected her own feelings of inadequacy in dealing with patients' non-physical needs of which spiritual needs are part.

3 Nurses indicated that they felt spiritual needs would become more apparent during crisis but gave no personal examples of crises they had faced to illustrate the point they were making. This may have been because they considered such experiences too personal to share. Alternatively they may never have personally encountered any crisis situations.

4 Nurses did not seem to demonstrate a personal search for meaning and purpose in their own lives e.g., they did not question why things had happened in their lives or in the lives of people close to them. If they had not experienced crises such questions may not have arisen.

In summary, it became apparent at interview that the three nurses who had indicated in the questionnaire that they had never identified a spiritual need, had actually done so. The reason given by them for this was connected with their belief system. Because they equated spiritual needs with religious needs, considered their beliefs private and themselves to be non-religious, they stated that they had not identified any religious needs.

Other characteristics of these nurses were noted by the researcher which may have been connected with their limited awareness of/ability to identify patients' spiritual needs and their tendency to give spiritual care at a superficial level. These included: their limited personal awareness of the spiritual dimension; their perceived inadequacy in helping patients with their spiritual needs; their apparent lack of life experiences such as crises which may have caused them to encounter spiritual needs personally and which may have been connected with their apparent lack of personal search for meaning. All of these factors could have stemmed ultimately from their belief system.

In addition these nurses differed in their grade and the type of ward and Health Board area in which they were working which may suggest that these factors were less important than the nurse's belief system and other personal characteristics in determining their identification of patients' spiritual needs.

Factors which appeared to prevent nurses from responding to patients' spiritual needs

Only one nurse in the sample had stated in the questionnaire that she had identified a spiritual need but did not indicate how she had responded. It emerged that she had experienced difficulty in answering the questions because she had not really thought about it before. This, coupled with lack of time, meant that she did not complete any of the other questions.

Through discussion, it emerged that she had identified a broad range of spiritual needs in patients (Figure 5.1) and had recognised them by patients communicating these directly, e.g., crying and by perceiving them at a deeper level herself, e.g., knowing the patient. She had responded by being personally involved to some extent, e.g., talking with patients, but she had referred patients' religious needs and those concerned with forgiveness to the clergy. On one occasion she had been involved at a deep personal level with a bereaved patient who was experiencing a situation she had recently encountered personally and had come to terms with. She evaluated the care she had given, in this instance, at the deepest level but experienced difficulty in evaluating in instances where patients were deaf or demented.

It would appear, in this case, that the life experience of the nurse was a factor which enabled her to give spiritual care. Other factors which interfered with the giving of spiritual care included deafness and dementia in patients for whom she was caring.

Other characteristics of this nurse were noted by the researcher as described below.

Although she did not consider herself a religious person she defined spiritual need in both religious and non-religious terms as indicated in her statement:

I feel it's between peoples' religious needs maybe and emotional needs which are surely tied up together.

and had identified both types of spiritual needs in patients. It would appear, therefore, that the spiritual needs she identified were in keeping with her perception of the term.

Furthermore, she stated that she felt unable to personally help patients with their religious needs because she was unsure of her own beliefs as illustrated in her statement:

I think...my bit wouldn't be...I don't think I would ever sort of talk about God to them. I would...talk about it in a more...emotional way rather than a religious way...probably the clergyman would talk about it more directly...because I'm so mixed up in my own religious beliefs...

Thus it appeared that this nurse's belief system, i.e., the uncertainty of her beliefs, influenced the way she responded to patients' spiritual needs, i.e., by referring to the clergy.

Although conclusions cannot be drawn from one nurse's experience, in this instance, lack of time and a limited awareness of the spiritual dimension in her own life, were factors given by this nurse for not having articulated the spiritual care she had given.

Further factors noted by the researcher which appeared to determine how spiritual care was given by this nurse included her perception of spiritual need, belief system, life experience and characteristics of patients which interfered with nurse-patient communication.

Factors which appeared to hinder the giving of effective spiritual care

None of the nurses in the sample considered the spiritual care given to have been totally ineffective. Three, however, considered it to have been more ineffective than effective because the patient's distressed condition remained largely unchanged.

They gave three reasons for this. First, they felt inadequate about personally helping patients with their spiritual needs because of their own lack of beliefs, fear of dealing with situations which they had personally not come to terms with or lack of experience in dealing with these needs. Second, they felt that lack of privacy and time meant that patients' spiritual needs were not adequately dealt with. Third, interventions which had been planned had not been carried out, e.g., the minister had not been contacted.

Factors which appeared to facilitate the giving of effective spiritual care

In the three instances where nurses had evaluated the spiritual care given as totally effective, the reason they gave was that previously noted distressing characteristics of the patient had been replaced by eustressing ones.

These nurses had recognised both types of spiritual needs, had given spiritual care at the deepest level and had not been hindered from doing so by any extraneous factors.

In conclusion, having explored with nurses some of their responses in the questionnaire, it seemed that the spiritual care given was determined by four main factors as outlined below.

1 *Smooth running of the nursing process in relation to spiritual care* (Figure 2.1). Effective spiritual care seemed to be facilitated when the nursing process flowed smoothly and when a change for the better in the patient's condition was noted. Ineffective spiritual care seemed to result when the nursing process was interrupted and there was little change in the patient's condition.

2 *Nurse related factors* The nurse's limited awareness of the spiritual dimension in her own life/lack of beliefs, lack of life experience or feelings of inadequacy in helping patients with their spiritual needs were factors which appeared to interfere with the giving of effective spiritual care.

3 *Patient related factors* In instances where patients were deaf, demented or unconscious it was difficult for nurses to identify their spiritual needs or evaluate the care given.

4 *Environmental factors* Lack of time and privacy interfered with the giving of spiritual care in some instances.

Factors noted by the researcher which appeared to have some bearing on the spiritual care nurses gave

When conducting the interviews it appeared to the researcher that the belief system of the nurse, her personal search for meaning and her perceptions of spiritual need and spiritual care were factors which seemed to determine the spiritual care she gave. Each factor is explored in turn.

Belief system

It seemed that nurses, who were not necessarily religious but demonstrated an awareness of God who was in ultimate control of their existence, were more aware of patients' spiritual needs and gave spiritual care at a deeper level than those who did not display these characteristics.

To enable the researcher to explore this hypothesis, nurses in the sample were classified according to whether or not they demonstrated these characteristics. These attributes were considered to be present if nurses made comments similar to those given below.

Comments indicating that nurses were aware of God in their own lives

...The need to think of things on a higher plane...having something to look up to, either a God or something else...

...deep down most...individuals want to please God...to be in harmonious relationship with the creator...and it's there whether they admit it or not.

...we all have this need...that there's somebody up there who's got the answer to the whole complex issues we all face.

When I was a child...I did have a warm feeling that God was there...but somewhere along the line, I don't have that warm feeling. I'd like to get it back again and I don't know how to get it back.

...you begin to think...a wee bit more deeply about what's maybe on the other side.

It was considered that nurses were not aware of God in their lives if they: made no comments about this or stated that they believed in the existence of God but did not relate it to their lives; indicated that they knew nothing about the spiritual dimension or had never really thought about it. Examples of comments indicative of the latter were:

To me spiritual is...religion...I really am not a very religious person myself so it would be a subject I wouldn't know what I was talking about really...I'm not going to be very good at this at all. I really don't know. It's something I really don't know anything about.

...my immediate reaction was good grief how am I going to fill it in (the questionnaire)...I put it away for quite some time and I got it out again...I found that really quite difficult. I haven't really thought about it...You're making me think of all sorts of things...I never bothered my head about...this is really rotten.

I don't think about it...I'm not religious...the good thing...was it made me think about it which I hadn't really thought about before.

Having set the above criteria and having previously ascertained the type of spiritual needs each nurse had identified and the level at which she had given spiritual care, it was possible to compare nurses' awareness of God with the level at which they gave spiritual care.

Comparison of the nurse's awareness of God with the level at which they gave spiritual care As Table 5.1 illustrates, nurses who demonstrated an awareness of God identified a broader range of spiritual needs and gave spiritual care at a deeper level than those who did not, i.e., they identified, responded and evaluated at a deeper level.

However, the nurse's awareness of God does not explain why some nurses who did not possess this attribute recognised both types of spiritual need at the deepest level and responded at the deepest level. It was decided, therefore, to look at how consistently individual nurses, who did not demonstrate an awareness of God, gave deep or superficial spiritual care.

Table 5.1 shows that, with the exception of nurse 6, all nurses who demonstrated an awareness of God consistently gave spiritual care at the deepest level, i.e., they had all recognised the spiritual need, responded to it and evaluated the effectiveness of this response at the deepest level. It emerged at interview that nurse 6 was unsure of her beliefs which may have explained why she was unable to respond to her patient's spiritual need at the deepest level.

Concerning the group of nurses which did not demonstrate an awareness of God, one third gave spiritual care consistently at the deepest level, i.e., recognised, responded and evaluated at the deepest level. Thus, although it would appear that those who demonstrated an awareness of God in their lives were more likely to consistently give spiritual care at a deep level than those who did not, it did not seem to be a necessary requirement.

Table 5.1
Type of spiritual needs identified and care given by nurses in relation to their personal awareness of God

Subject No.	Aware of God						Unaware of God					
	1	2	3	4	5	6	7	8	9	10	11	12
Type of needs identified	1+2	2	1+2	1+2	2	2	3	3	3	1+2	2	1+2
Level at which needs recognised	ab	b	b	ab	ab	b	a	a	b	ab	b	a
Level of response	o	mo	mo	mo	mno	n	m	mn	m	mno	mo	mo
Level of evaluation	yz	xyz	xyz	xyz	xyz	z	y	y	xyz	xyz	yz	xy

KEY Terms as defined in Figure 5.1

Type of spiritual needs identified:
1 = Type 1 needs   2 = Type 2 needs
3 = stated initially that they had not identified a spiritual need but at interview it emerged that they had identified religious needs only

Level at which spiritual needs were recognised:
a = 1st level   b = 2nd level

Level at which nurses responded to patients' spiritual needs:
m = 1st level   n = 2nd level   o = 3rd level

Level at which nurses evaluated spiritual care given:
x = 1st level   y = 2nd level   z = 3rd level

Source: Author's own

Personal search for meaning

It seemed that nurses who appeared to be searching for meaning in their own lives were more aware of patients' spiritual needs and gave care at a deeper level than those who did not. Nurses were classified, by the researcher, according to whether or not they demonstrated search for meaning. It was assumed they demonstrated this characteristic if they made comments similar to those listed below:

> ...what meaning you make of your life...and how you conduct yourself so that your conscience is leading you so that in the end you maybe hopefully go to heaven or something similar.

> I think the meaning of life varies through your life. There are different facets to it...everything in life gives life meaning.

As stated above, it was assumed that nurses were not searching for meaning in their lives if they made no reference to this throughout the interview. Having classified nurses in this way, it was possible to compare the two groups as shown in Table 5.2.

Nurses who demonstrated the need to find meaning and purpose in their own lives seemed to identify non-religious needs whereas those who did not display this characteristic appeared to identify mainly religious needs or both types of needs. The former group, however, seemed to respond and evaluate at a deeper level than the latter group.

It would seem, therefore, that although nurses who demonstrated no personal need to find meaning in their lives appeared to identify a wider variety of spiritual needs than those demonstrating this characteristic, the latter group seemed to give spiritual care at the deepest level.

Nurses' perceptions of spiritual need and spiritual care

It seemed that the type of spiritual needs nurses identified and the care they gave corresponded with their perceptions of these terms, e.g., nurses who defined spiritual need in religious and broader terms would identify both types of need in practice and those who considered it the nurse's role to respond to both types of need in practice would do so.

In order to explore this observation, nurses' definitions of spiritual need and spiritual care were compared with the spiritual needs they identified and the responses they gave respectively. The results are presented in Table 5.3.

Table 5.2
Type of spiritual needs identified and care given by nurses in relation to their personal search for meaning

	Search for meaning							No search for meaning					
Subject No.	1	2	3	4	5	6		1	2	3	4	5	6
Type of needs ident- ified	1+2	2	2	1+2	2	2		1+2	1	1	1+2	1+2	1+2
Level at which needs rec- ognised	ab	b	b	ab	ab	b		a	a	ab	ab	a	b
Level of response	o	mo	mo	mo	mno	n		m	mn	m	mno	mo	mo
Level of evalua- tion	yz	yz	xyz	xyz	xyz	z		y	y	xyz	xyz	xy	xyz

KEY as in Table 5.1

Source: Author's own

As shown in Table 5.3, the spiritual needs identified and the care given by nurses seemed, on the whole, to correspond with their definitions of these terms. However, the needs identified and care given by nurses may ultimately be more connected with the spiritual needs the nurse herself had experienced and the extent to which she had come to terms with certain spiritual issues e.g., death, dying. Her personal experience may trace back eventually to her fundamental beliefs about life, death, her life experience and the extent to which she was self-actualised.

In conclusion, within the sample, it appeared that the belief system of the nurse, her personal search for meaning and her perception of spiritual need and spiritual care were factors which may have influenced which spiritual needs she recognised and the spiritual care she gave.

Table 5.3
A comparison of nurses' definitions of spiritual need and spiritual care with their professed practice

Sub-ject No.	Definition of spiritual need	Spiritual needs identified
1	Religious. spiritual needs. religion.	Initially stated had not identified any spiritual Later religious : to practise
2	Religious + non-religious. to pray.	Initially stated had not identified any spiritual needs. Later religious: for priest prior to death,
3	Religious.	Initially stated had not identified anys piritual needs. Later religious: for mass.
4	Religious + non-religious.	Religious: for communion. Non-religious: for love.
5	Religious + non-religious.	Religious: for reassurance that going to heaven. Non-religious: relief from fear of dying.
6	Religious + non-religious.	Non-religious: to be prepared for death.
7	Religious + non-religious.	Religious: to see Rabbi. Non-religious: for love.
8	Religious + non-religious + deeper God related.	Non-religious: for peace.
9	Religious + deeper God related.	Deeper God related: to put things right with God. Non-religious: to be prepared for death.
10	Religious + non-religious + deeper God related.	Religious: for sacraments. Non-religious: to be known. Deeper God related: for reconciliation with God.

Sub- ject No.	Definition of spiritual need	Spiritual needs identified
11	Religious + non-religious + deeper God related.	Non-religious: to come to terms with death.
12	Religious + deeper God related.	Non-religious: to be free from fear.

Sub- ject No.	Definition of spiritual care	Response to patients' spiritual needs
1	Don't know.	Allowed religious representative access.
2	To recognise a spiritual need and refer.	Recognised need and contacted clergy.
3	Care given by clergy.	Contacted clergy.
4	To refer with religious needs + respond personally to non-religious needs.	Referred religious needs + issue concerning need for forgiveness. Responded personally to other needs, e.g., showed love by giving good care.
5	To refer with some religious rituals + respond person- ally with some religious and non-religious needs.	Responded personally to religious needs, e.g., read Bible, pray with patient + non-religious needs, e.g., 'being with' patient.
6	To refer with religious needs + respond personally to non-religious	Referred needs related to death and the after-life that had not come to terms with herself. Responded personally with some issues concerning death, e.g., talked with patient about

156

Sub-ject No.	Definition of spiritual care	Response to patients' spiritual needs
	+ some religious needs.	religion + non-religious issues.
7	To refer with religious needs + respond personally to non-religious needs	Referred religious issues, e.g., contacted Rabbi + helped with non-religious needs e.g., showed love through touch.
8	To respond personally to non-religious + deeper God related needs + refer with rituals.	Responded to non-religious needs e.g., 'being with' patient.
9	To respond personally to some religious needs + refer with others.	Responded to non-religious needs, e.g., listened + referred religious needs.
10	To respond to all needs except some religious rituals.	Responded to: deeper God related needs, e.g., shared own experiences of God; non-religious needs, e.g., listened and gave hope. Referred sacraments.
11	To respond to all needs except some religious rituals.	Responded to non-religious needs, e.g., 'being with', prayed with patient.
12	To respond to all needs except some religious rituals.	Responded to non-religious needs, e.g., listened.

Source: Author's own

Exploration of the characteristics of nurses in relation to the level of spiritual care given

An alternative measure employed to identify factors which may have influenced the spiritual care given by nurses was to look at the characteristics displayed by those who consistently gave spiritual care either at a deep or a superficial level. These are discussed in turn below. In addition, demographic information about each respondent is given. It was felt that any differences in characteristics identified between the two groups may point to factors which could have influenced how spiritual care was given. Again researcher bias was acknowledged in the analysis.

Characteristics of nurses who gave the most comprehensive spiritual care

Nurses were considered to have given the most comprehensive spiritual care if in every example cited by them they recognised, responded and evaluated at the deepest level.

Four nurses had given care in this way. The transcripts of their interviews were re-read and the following common characteristics were noted. All comments refer to the four nurses.

They seemed to be particularly sensitive/perceptive This is demonstrated by the following examples of comments they made:

Nurse 1 S/N, Single, 20-29 yrs old, 6-10 yrs experience, long term care ward, Dumfries & Galloway, R/C.

> ...its like when you say spiritual I can feel it. I can't explain it...but I can feel it...

> ...it's like an unseen bond between her and her daughter...something in her daughter just isn't right...I really can't explain it...I can actually feel that she's not satisfied but I can't explain to you what it is that's missing...

Nurse 2 C/N, Single, 20-29 yrs old, 6-10 yrs experience, long term care, Argyll & Clyde, C/S.

> I knew she was going to die quite a wee while before anyone else suspected it. I thought she's not going to come out of this.

> ...it wasn't anything she said...attitudes. I think it was more her face actually....her eyes...very expressive eyes...mirroring what's going

on...sometimes she'd put out her hand...and take hold of my hand...you got a transfer.

...there's a kind of radiation comes from people...if you touch them you can feel the life force going through the body...many's a time I've taken somebody's BP and pulse...been within normal parameters and I have questioned the vitality of that individual...and ultimately something has happened to prove me right.

(speaking of her daughter who had anorexia)...this particular night...she was lying next to me...I could feel the life force that was dominant in me and not in her...I thought is there no way I can transfer some of this from me to her...I began to really think about it and will it to happen...I felt a tingling along the parts of my body that were in contact with her...after that there was a subtle difference in her condition...you felt her energy levels rising and within a relatively short time...she went and picked up an apple and began to eat it.

Nurse 3 S/N, married, 30-39 yrs old, 11-25 yrs experience, varied ward, Argyll and Clyde, R/C.

I would say it was more than that...the spark within her was probably kindled...

...she was unhappy...her facial expression, her conversation...the necessity for alcohol...I believe she wanted an escape from reality if you will...

At that time I felt her spirit needed fed.

Hopefully we're giving them a tomorrow to look forward to...what is typically seen in bad geriatric care are little faces that have no tomorrow and some of them will even wish they had no tomorrow...showing that you can identify to their true selves...a smile...it's almost as if the person inside there is saying thank you you understand...

Nurse 4 S/N, widow, 50-59 yrs old, 11-25 yrs experience, long term care, Lothian, C/S, beginning psychiatric training.

...sometimes if they're very uneasy and just unhappy in themselves...

I hope mental training will help with this to learn to really listen to what they're saying inside as much as outside...

They demonstrated an awareness of the spiritual dimension in everyday living
These nurses seemed to be deeply aware of the spiritual dimension in their daily lives and appeared to have thought it through. This was indicated by the fact that they had a lot to say on the subject and related the spiritual dimension to all aspects of life e.g., world events, re-incarnation, death and dying, psychopaths, appreciation of scenery.

They demonstrated an awareness of God who was in ultimate control of their existence Although not necessarily religious, these nurses seemed to be aware of God as illustrated in the following extracts taken from the transcripts:

Nurse 1
...because I have some belief myself I maybe just find it difficult to believe that somebody has absolutely no belief in anything.

...I believe in a soul...we've all got a soul...although you could have a psychological need met...it may not have reached your soul...

Nurse 2
...what I understand with the real core meaning of spirituality is a need for a higher spiritual presence than man or any other living creature...it basically arises from a source within us, the soul if you want to call it that...there is something deep within the core of every individual.

I'm not a member of a particular religious group...if I was going to describe myself...certainly not an atheist and I don't think agnostic really fits me...there's something missing with all the ...religious dogma...

...if you didn't have any spirituality yourself how could you possibly get on to the same wavelength...it's all to do with wavelength...

Nurse 3
If I hadn't been a Christian nurse...the situation may have gone unnoticed...(it was) significant for me because I'm a Christian...my child had just made her first Holy Communion...and I showed photographs to the patient who said to me 'well of course that's not part of my life any more'...of course immediately as a Christian I had to say to her that everyone was deserving...you may feel at the time there was an intervention of the Holy Spirit...

Nurse 4

I think God is a being whom we can know personally...I think too life after death is a very definite thing...

I would say that the whole of our being is a spiritual need...the whole of life is related to God.

They appeared willing to give of themselves to others   These nurses were actively involved in helping patients with their spiritual needs at a deep personal level themselves, as illustrated by the following extracts from the transcripts:

Nurse 1

It's a physical thing as well...I strongly believe in physical contact...reassurance might only be holding someone's hand...giving them a cuddle...just being there...sitting and talking...

...what you believe and what they believe might be totally incompatible...you don't have to be of the same religion to provide them with the reassurance they want. As long as you're not frightened to speak to them about it.

Nurse 2

...when she did die I called out the doctor and I said to him...'in the bad old days of nursing someone would have been found to sit with that patient' and he said 'oh but she wasn't aware' I said 'well we don't actually know that whether she was aware or not I feel strongly that no-one should die alone in a hospital

...my sister is actually dying at the moment of a malignant brain tumour...when I speak to her I don't know if they've done this or not (tell her her diagnosis)...it makes it very difficult for me...I would like to be able to...sit with her and talk it through...want to be honest with her...I want to talk to her on a deeper emotional plane and I just can't

Nurse 3

...it's something that you feel is personal to yourself and to a relationship with yourself and your patient...it's something you're aware that you are giving different patients. You know that you have something to offer the patient at that particular level...it's targeting the self of a person...it's seeing them as absolutely unique...

161

(talking of her relationship with the patient)...this is what I represent and anything that that represents I'm here to give you...(regardless of my) circumstances...I am the nurse for you...

Nurse 4

I would feel able to be me with that person...inside I would be praying...sometimes I have a little booklet...I think you have to be sensitive...I do consciously commit them to God as often as I can...

They appeared to be searching for meaning and purpose in their own lives
This characteristic is illustrated in the following extracts:

Nurse 1

...I feel sometimes...I maybe don't have strong beliefs myself...I perhaps don't believe that life probably ends when you die. I think life as we know it does but I'm not sure...

(talking of the need for reassurance and guidance)...I think it comes sporadically in life...it's not always when something terrible is happening...you might be the same as you were physically 6 weeks ago but emotionally you're on a low...

Nurse 2

...you might start with a particular ideology...then towards the end of your life you realise there is a gap - I feel it myself...we all have this need that there is somebody up there who's got the answer to the whole complex issues that we all face...

...(speaking of her sister who was dying) explore what might be ahead for both of us...I'm 57...nobody knows how long they've got...you begin to think a wee bit more deeply about what's maybe on the other side...

Nurse 3

...perhaps she was led to her spiritual awakening through this very difficult physical situation...

...I like reading it (philosophy)...I pick it up and I read it and say thats marvellous..fascinating..fabulous ideas...

Nurse 4

..they're very deep thoughtful questions (asked at interview)...it'll make me think for years.

162

...he (God) can give us a whole purpose in living and a whole purpose in what we're doing and relationships with other people...He can meet our need for forgiveness...freedom from guilt...

They shared of life experiences and what they had learned from these
Throughout the interviews these nurses made constant reference to personal life events such as crises and shared what they had learned from these experiences. Examples of this are given below:

Nurse 1
...I tended to look back through my nursing career and I think...I'm much better prepared...I think my patients have prepared me...I think because...I've gone through bereavement...more than I had when I was even 10 years ago when I was 20. There's been a lot more bereavement in the family and all the rest of it and I've coped with it. If you're helping relatives it's easier to know what they want...you've been through the process...you know what they're going through...you're better prepared for facing the people that you're going to be helping through it...

...I expect the clergy to have stronger beliefs than I do...I may not be so reticent to do that in the future...because I feel I know more about it...I'm more experienced...

Nurse 2
...(speaking of patient who was dying) I don't know if I could say empathy because I've never actually been dying...I tried to feel as much understanding as I could considering I hadn't actually been in the situation myself...

...I know how I feel since my husband died...the lack of the physical presence of another human being...leaves a big gap...just the feeling that there is another person that cares enough about you with   all your failings, to sit with you...

Nurse 3
(when asked if she would feel able to personally help a patient of a different faith) ...well in my instance having married a Hindu it would present no difficulty at all.

Nurse 4
...you knew what they were feeling...my husband died suddenly so in that sense...you just seem to appreciate what she was going through...

163

Characteristics of nurses who gave the most superficial spiritual care

It was considered that nurses had given the most superficial spiritual care if they did not recognise and respond or evaluate at the deepest level in any patient examples cited by them. Two nurses gave care in this way. Following examination of their transcripts, they appeared to demonstrate the following characteristics.

They did not seem notably sensitive/perceptive to patients' spiritual needs
This was the general impression given by statements similar to the following:

Nurse 1   S/N, married, 21-29 yrs old, <1 yr in practice, long term care, Dumfries & Galloway, no religious affiliation.

> We ask them their religion...but it doesn't go much further than that...you step back...

> It would be up to them really to let you in...they wanted certain surroundings...privacy...certain people there and they got that but I don't know about their...needs...the rest was up to them...

Nurse 2   C/N, married, over 60 yrs of age, over 26 yrs experience, long term care, Argyll & Clyde, C/S.

> (when asked if she thought some nurses could give spiritual care)...Oh aye there's lots. I'm sure there are and do it

> (when asked if she considered herself in that category) I don't know, I'd do anything a patient asked me to.

They did not seem to have much idea about or to have given much thought to the spiritual dimension before   This was indicated by the following examples of statements made by them:

Nurse 1
I really am not a very religious person myself so it would be a subject I wouldn't know what I was talking about really...how can I say anybody has or hasn't got spiritual needs.

It's maybe people...look for reassurance that they don't think anybody else can give them...a magical sort of untouchable sort...something with more importance to it... (when asked what the thing with more importance was)

...I don't know. A power, I can't describe it...I just don't see it as part of our work...what spiritual care can nurses give I mean we care for them physically and mentally...I just can't see that we can...

Nurse 2
I had to read it over and over again (the questionnaire) and then I brought it home.

(When asked what spiritual needs patients might have) ...well I'm sure most people say 'God help me' or I don't know I'm probably on the wrong track...I feel that they'd have to have friends...they would need some help but I don't know what type...I don't know...

They considered their beliefs to be a private and personal matter Statements made by nurses which alerted the researcher to the fact that they considered their beliefs a private matter were:

Nurse 1
...it's something too personal...I feel you're going into ground that you've got no right to be in...I would hate anybody....wanting to get that close to me...I'm a very guarded person..."

Nurse 2
I believe in God...I haven't been to church for a few years....at first I thought it's really a private sort of thing...to discuss anything like that with a patient.

They seemed reluctant to share of themselves at a deep level when giving spiritual care The above characteristic is captured in the following extracts:

Nurse 1
(talking of meeting of patients' spiritual needs)...they might go to their family...people close to them...members of their religion but I don't think we're that close...I don't think we should get that close...I think it's too personal...if you get that close you get too involved...maybe I observe from a distance..(When asked if the nurse could be involved in spiritual care) ...well if she felt she could...help...that's fair enough but I personally don't...you should be your own motivator, if you want to do it you should do it. I don't think it should be taught. I don't think you could.

Nurse 2
..I felt I couldn't give a lot of spiritual need to a patient except through the clergy...

They did not appear to demonstrate a personal search for meaning and purpose in their own lives Nurse 2 gave no indication at any point in the interview of a personal search for meaning in her life. Nurse 1 acknowledged that life must have meaning but appeared unsure about it as indicated by her statement:

There's a meaning in life...there must be motivation of some sort...I really don't know. It's just something   I really don't know anything about...

They did not share any life experiences from which they had learned Nurse 1 said she felt spiritual needs would arise in crisis but gave no personal examples of crisis in her own life. When asked if she had ever contacted the clergy on behalf of a patient she replied:

No...I've never been involved with that.

Nurse 2 said she felt guilty about not going to church and about not having spent time with her mother before she died. She dealt with her guilt by asking God to forgive her and would not have felt comfortable talking to the minister or anyone else about it. Thus her actions were in keeping with her belief system, i.e., that this was a private and personal matter.

In conclusion, it would appear, from the limited number of nurses studied, that the following characteristics of nurses were conducive to the giving of spiritual care at a deep level:

1 Awareness of the spiritual dimension in everyday living.
2 Awareness of God.
3 Personal search for meaning and purpose in life.
4 Having experience and learned from life events, e.g., crises.
5 Willingness to give of self to others.
6 Sensitivity/perceptivity.

Nurses who gave spiritual care superficially either did not demonstrate the above characteristics or did so to a lesser degree. Nurses who gave spiritual care deeply or superficially varied in their grade, geographical location, type of ward, age, marital status, religious affiliation and length of time in practice. This suggests that the personal characteristics identified in this chapter may be more instrumental in determining the spiritual care nurses gave than those previously identified through the cross-tabulation of variables.

17 Summary and conclusions

Although it is not possible to make generalisations from such a small sample, the semi-structured interviews conducted with twelve nurses nevertheless highlighted a number of factors which may have influenced the spiritual care they gave. In addition, the findings provide possible clues as to factors which may have influenced the care given by nurses in the larger sample, although this cannot be assumed.

Five main factors, similar to those identified by Hockey (1979) (Figure 2.2), appeared to influence the spiritual care that this sample of nurses gave and are summarised in Figure 5.4. These were related to the nurse, patient, other professionals, environment and operation of the nursing process. Each factor is discussed below.

First, concerning the nurse, it seemed that nurses who demonstrated a personal search for meaning in their own lives, although they identified a narrower range of spiritual needs, gave spiritual care at a deeper level than those who did not demonstrate this characteristic. As search for meaning is a spiritual concern (Part 1), this finding may be directly related to the belief system of the nurse which also seemed to be connected with the spiritual care she gave. The belief system of the nurse was similarly identified in other studies as a factor influencing the general care (Forrest, 1989, Samarel, 1991) and spiritual care (Piles, 1986) nurses gave.

Initially it appeared that nurses who claimed religious affiliation were better able to identify patients' spiritual needs than those who did not (Part 4, Section 12). The interviews revealed, however, that the nurse's personal awareness of the spiritual dimension and of God, regardless of whether these were expressed through religious means, may have been more important in determining the spiritual care she gave. This is illustrated by the fact that nurses who demonstrated these characteristics identified a broad range of spiritual needs and give spiritual care at a deep level, whereas those who showed limited

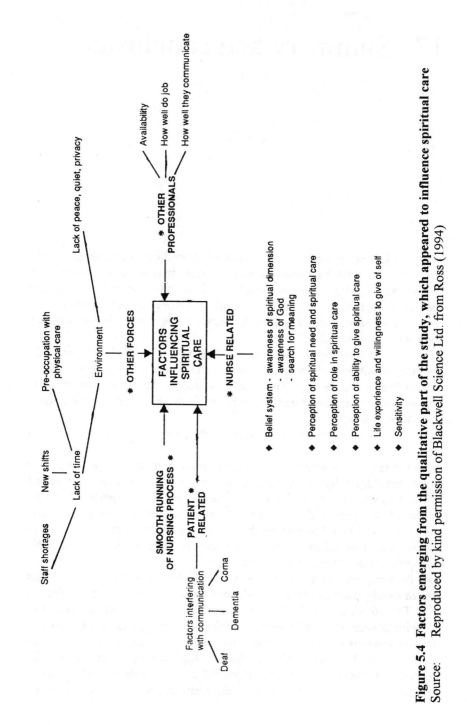

Figure 5.4 Factors emerging from the qualitative part of the study, which appeared to influence spiritual care
Source: Reproduced by kind permission of Blackwell Science Ltd. from Ross (1994)

awareness of the spiritual dimension and were unsure of their beliefs found it difficult to give spiritual care.

Statistical analysis in Part 4 (Section 12) revealed that C/N's identified more spiritual needs than S/N's. It was suggested that nurses who had gone through certain life experiences and hence were more mature, may have been better able to identify patients' spiritual needs than those who were less mature. The finding from the interviews suggests that the maturity/life experience factor is perhaps more important than the grade of the nurse in determining the spiritual care given, however, this could not be explained by the fact that C/N's were older or more clinically experienced.

For instance, nurses seemed to be able to personally respond to spiritual needs which they had themselves encountered. This may explain why they seemed to identify spiritual needs and give spiritual care in keeping with their perceptions of these terms and why some nurses were willing to be personally involved in giving spiritual care whereas others felt inadequate in this respect. In a similar vein, Forrest (1989) found that the nurse's own experience affected her caring and Samarel (1991) reported how nurses who had personally come to terms with death were able to help terminally ill patients.

Furthermore, the nurse's perception of her role appeared to influence the care she gave e.g., nurses who did not consider spiritual care their duty did not give it. This is consistent with the findings of Highfield and Cason (1983), Hitchens (1988) and Piles (1986). In a similar vein, Forrest (1989) found that the nurse's own experience affected her caring and Samarel (1991) reported how nurses who had personally come to terms with death were able to help terminally ill patients. Moreover, the nature of the nurse appeared to influence the spiritual care she gave in that those nurses who were particularly sensitive people seemed to identify the broadest range of spiritual needs and give spiritual care at the deepest level.

Additionally, the nurse's grade and the type of ward and geographical area in which she was working, (factors found to be associated with the identification of spiritual needs by nurses in Part 4), did not seem to affect the level of spiritual care she gave. This further supports the suggestion that the personal characteristics of the nurse are perhaps more important than these other factors in determining the spiritual care given. The influence of grade, ward type and geographical location in the giving of spiritual care cannot be ruled out, however, further research would be required to ascertain this and to determine if any of the reasons offered by nurses as possible explanations were valid.

Second, the nature of the patient's condition seemed to influence the spiritual care nurses gave. It seemed to make it difficult for nurses to give spiritual care if patients were demented, deaf, comatosed or unresponsive for whatever other reason. This was similarly borne out by Samarel's (1991) study and may explain why nurses working on non-varied wards reported identifying fewer spiritual needs than those on varied wards (Part 4, Section 12).

Third, the unavailability of, inadequate care given by and lack of communication with other professionals such as clergy and environmental factors such as lack of time, peace, quiet and privacy were factors nurses stated interfered with them giving spiritual care. Lack of time was also a factor identified by other researchers which interfered with the giving of care in general (Forrest, 1991; Samarel, 1991) and with spiritual care in particular (Piles, 1986).

Finally, in more general terms, it appeared from exploring with nurses the spiritual care they gave, that none applied the nursing process to spiritual care and that any factor which interfered with the smooth running of this process (Figure 2.1) delayed or prevented effective spiritual care from being given.

Part Six
CONCLUSIONS

18 Overview of the study

The purpose of this Part is to give an overview of the study and its main findings before discussing their implications. Tentative suggestions for nursing practice are then given and topics for further research are proposed.

Having illustrated that the spiritual dimension can influence health, well-being and quality of life, it was shown that spiritual care should be part of the nurse's role. However, guidelines for its practice were absent in the nursing literature and nothing was known about how British nurses perceived their role in this aspect of care (Part 1).

A conceptual framework for giving spiritual care based on the Nursing Process was, therefore, proposed by the author (Part 2). It was recognised, however, that there is currently a lack of knowledge to enable the conceptual framework to be enacted and furthermore it would require to be tested. As outlined in Part 3, the study aims were twofold and a dual approach, which blended both quantitative (Part 4) and qualitative (Part 5) methods was adopted to address these aims. Every method has its pros and cons thus use of a dual approach limited the study in a number of ways.

Perhaps one of the study's main weaknesses lies in the fact that the sample of nurses responding (n=685) may not have been representative of the population (n=1170). In addition not all Health Boards were included. It cannot be assumed, therefore, that the way in which the sample of nurses stated they perceived spiritual need and spiritual care and gave this care in practice, was indicative of the population, or the same group of nurses working in Scotland as a whole or any other part of the country. Additionally, the findings relate only to nurses working on care of the elderly wards. There is suggestion that spiritual needs may be more prevalent in acute settings (Part 4), however further research would be required to ascertain this. The findings cannot, therefore, be generalised to nurses working in settings other than care of the elderly. Moreover, it was assumed that what nurses said they did was what they actually did, however this may not have been the case.

The sample of nurses from which information was obtained with regard to factors influencing spiritual care was very small (n=12) and selected on the basis of set criteria. It cannot be assumed therefore that the factors identified as apparently influential in the giving of spiritual care were the same for the larger sample (n=685), the population or any other group.

Finally, although measures were employed to minimise its effects, the study is further limited by researcher bias. This is acknowledged particularly in relation to the categorisation of responses to open questions, selection of the sample for interviews and in the analysis of the transcripts.

Given the above limitations, the results, a synopsis of which is now given, can only be taken as indicative of the sample.

The first part of the study described how 685 nurses working in care of the elderly settings in twelve Health Boards in Scotland perceived spiritual need and spiritual care and how they gave this care (Part 4). The majority of nurses said they had identified a spiritual need at some point in their practice. Collectively as a group they perceived the concept in terms of the individual's need for: belief and faith; for peace and comfort; to give and receive love and forgiveness; for meaning, purpose and fulfilment; for hope and creativity. They had a propensity, however, to view spiritual need in religious terms. They recognised patients' spiritual needs mainly through non-verbal/indirect verbal cues patients displayed.

Although the majority of nurses considered it their shared responsibility to respond to patients' spiritual needs and some did so personally, over half preferred to refer them to others, mainly the clergy, possibly because they felt inadequate about personally responding.

Most nurses evaluated the care which had been given positively and did so through observing non-verbal/indirect verbal cues patients displayed. As Table 4.13 shows, the cues nurses used in evaluating were the opposite of those which had alerted them to patients' needs (Table 4.11).

In the second part of the study a variety of analyses were employed and five factors, similar to those cited by Hockey (1989) (Figure 2.2), were identified which appeared to influence the spiritual care nurses gave (Parts 4 and 5). These related to the nurse, patient, other professionals, environment and smooth running of the nursing process.

Statistical analysis in the larger sample (n=685) revealed that charge nurses claiming religious affiliation seemed better able to identify patients' spiritual needs than staff nurses who claimed none (Part 4). Based on the smaller sample (n=12), more in-depth analysis suggested that, rather than grade and religious affiliation, personal characteristics of the nurse were perhaps more important in determining their giving of spiritual care. Although further research would be required to clarify this it seemed that nurses who demonstrated an awareness of the spiritual dimension in their own lives; were personally searching for meaning; had experienced crises; perceived spiritual care as part of their role; and were particularly sensitive/perceptive people, were able to identify a broader range of spiritual needs and give spiritual care at a deeper level than those who did not demonstrate these characteristics (Part 5).

Second, any factors in the patient's condition which interfered with nurse-patient communication seemed to make it difficult for nurses to identify spiritual needs and give spiritual care (Parts 4 and 5).

Also, the unavailability of, inadequate care given by and lack of communication with other professionals, particularly the clergy, together with environmental factors such as lack of time, peace, quiet and privacy seemed to hinder some nurses from giving spiritual care (Parts 4 and 5). Concerning environmental factors, although explanations were suggested for the association between ward type and the identification of spiritual needs by nurses in the larger sample, none could be offered for the association of the latter with the geographical location of nurses (Part 4).

Finally, it was suggested in Part 2 that the best way of ensuring that patients' spiritual needs were met was by giving care systematically using the nursing process. From the smaller sample (n=12), there was evidence to suggest that the Nursing Process may not be applied to spiritual care (Part 5), and that any of the above mentioned factors could interfere with the smooth running of that process.

As discussed above, because of the nature of the study, the findings cannot be generalised, their implications can only be tentative and suggestions rather than recommendations for practice only can be given. These are discussed in Chapter 19.

19 Implications

Although the majority of nurses seemed able to identify patients' spiritual needs, on closer scrutiny they may have performed this function less well than the results of the study indicate.

First it was not possible to ascertain to what extent they had identified patients' spiritual needs.

Second, as suggested in Part 4, the proportion of nurses considering spiritual care not part of their role may have been higher in the population than the results of the study indicated.

Third, the fact that nurses seemed to define spiritual need in religious terms, together with the fact that the smaller sample seemed to identify spiritual needs and give care in keeping with their perceptions of these terms, implies that patients' religious needs may be more readily identified than other spiritual needs they may have or that spiritual needs are most commonly expressed in religious terms. Also, if nurses considered spiritual and psychological needs to be synonymous, they may ignore spiritual interventions in helping patients who were, for instance, struggling to find meaning in their illness. Furthermore, there was suggestion that the identification of patients' spiritual needs may depend on the sensitivity of the nurse. The implications of these findings are that for some patients all/some of their spiritual needs may go unrecognised or may be inadequately or inappropriately dealt with thus hindering them from attaining an optimum level of spiritual well-being and overall state of health, the importance of which is illustrated in Figure 1.7.

Whether they did not consider spiritual care part of their role or felt inadequate about giving it, the fact that, in general, nurses did not feel personally able to respond to patients' spiritual needs implies that patients' may have experienced delay in having these needs met or that their needs may not have been met at all, or only partially met, e.g., in the case of referral. Referral in itself may not be detrimental to ensuring that action is taken to meet patients' spiritual needs as ultimately what matters is that patients' needs are met. However, in the real world the referral process, whether to other nurses, clergy or others, may not operate efficiently and may therefore interrupt the nursing process resulting in delay/prevention of patients' having their spiritual needs met. This may happen for a number of reasons as outlined in Figure 6.1. It should be noted that the situation described in the figure is not as clear cut as it appears but is presented in this way for illustration purposes. Furthermore, even if the referral process operated smoothly, it would still introduce discontinuity of care.

On the whole, nurses considered the spiritual care given to have been effective and reached this conclusion through re-assessing the patient's condition. Some nurses, however, made this assumption on the basis that an event had occurred, e.g., the minister had visited. In such cases it is possible that the patient's need may not have been met but, because the nurse assumed it had been met, alternative interventions may not have been instigated.

The expectation is that the broader the range of spiritual needs nurses can identify and respond to at the deepest level, the more likely patients' spiritual needs will be met and an optimum level of total health, well-being and quality of life facilitated (Figure 5.2). It would appear, therefore, that nurses who were themselves spiritually aware, were personally searching for meaning in life; had experienced crises; perceived spiritual care as part of their role and were particularly sensitive/perceptive people, would be best able to operate in this way. This implies, however, that patients being cared for by nurses not in possession of these qualities may not have their spiritual needs well attended to. It also raises the question as to whether or not all nurses can be expected to identify a broad range of spiritual needs and give spiritual care at a deep level. If not, perhaps nurses who could would be over burdened. Furthermore whether or not patients' spiritual needs were met would depend on the efficiency of the referral process.

Moreover, the fact that nurses found it difficult to identify spiritual needs in patients suffering from conditions such as dementia, deafness etc., implies that it may be difficult for nurses to identify spiritual needs in patients suffering from any conditions interfering with nurse-patient communication. Although the list of such patients is endless examples include those afflicted with: aphasia; dysphasia; loss of affect because of depression, drug therapy, CVA, institutionalisation; confusion, whether induced by drugs, infection or other causes as well as those who are unconscious. The implication is that for all these patients their spiritual needs may not be recognised.

Additionally, patients who are highly physically dependent or situated in wards which are short staffed, noisy, lacking in privacy, which operate new shift patterns or where there is poor collaboration with the clergy, may not have their spiritual needs well attended to.

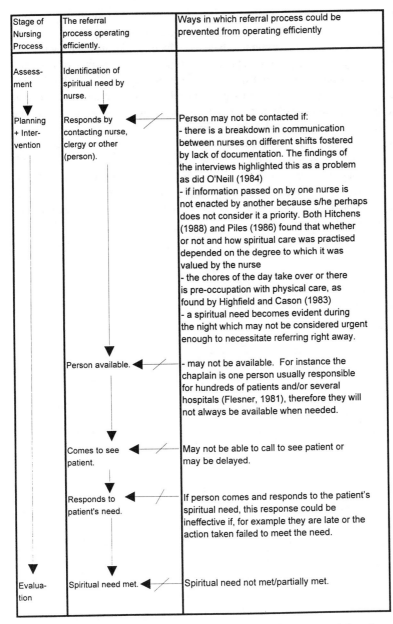

Stage of Nursing Process	The referral process operating efficiently.	Ways in which referral process could be prevented from operating efficiently
Assess-ment	Identification of spiritual need by nurse.	
Planning + Inter-vention	Responds by contacting nurse, clergy or other (person).	Person may not be contacted if: - there is a breakdown in communication between nurses on different shifts fostered by lack of documentation. The findings of the interviews highlighted this as a problem as did O'Neill (1984) - if information passed on by one nurse is not enacted by another because s/he perhaps does not consider it a priority. Both Hitchens (1988) and Piles (1986) found that whether or not and how spiritual care was practised depended on the degree to which it was valued by the nurse - the chores of the day take over or there is pre-occupation with physical care, as found by Highfield and Cason (1983) - a spiritual need becomes evident during the night which may not be considered urgent enough to necessitate referring right away.
	Person available.	- may not be available. For instance the chaplain is one person usually responsible for hundreds of patients and/or several hospitals (Flesner, 1981), therefore they will not always be available when needed.
	Comes to see patient.	May not be able to call to see patient or may be delayed.
	Responds to patient's need.	If person comes and responds to the patient's spiritual need, this response could be ineffective if, for example they are late or the action taken failed to meet the need.
Evalua-tion	Spiritual need met.	Spiritual need not met/partially met.

Figure 6.1   Possible pitfalls of referring patients' spiritual needs to others

Source: Author's own

Finally, as a general but nevertheless important point, it would appear that nurses may not be used to applying the nursing process to spiritual care and also that there are many potential factors which could interfere with the smooth running of this process. This could result in discontinuity of care and delay or prevention in the giving of effective spiritual care. Such an outcome would, therefore, be detrimental to patients who had spiritual needs in that they would be hindered from attaining an optimum level of spiritual and hence overall well-being as discussed in Part 1 (Figure 1.7).

It could be argued that whenever such factors prevent spiritual needs from being recognised, that a situation of nurse induced iatrogenesis (Illich, 1975) emerges in that the very state of health which nursing aims to promote is hindered by its own structure and the environment in which it functions. For instance, administrative constraints may mean that nurses do not have the time to give the care they would like.

20 Suggestions for practice

Given the limitations of this descriptive study, firm recommendations for practice are not warranted, therefore, tentative suggestions only are made.

It would appear that if the spiritual needs of patients are to be identified and met and patients are consequently to be assisted to achieve an optimum level of health and well-being it is important that nurses are able to give spiritual care systematically.

There is indication that some nurses need to be made aware that spiritual care is part of their duty, whilst for others their concept of spiritual need requires to be broadened. As stated in the guidelines for nurse education (Part 1) nurses would probably benefit from some form of teaching on spiritual care in their basic education. However, the way in which spiritual care could best be taught is not clear. Formal teaching could include topics such as description and definition of the spiritual dimension, spiritual needs and spiritual care in the broadest terms; the influence of the spiritual dimension on health and therefore the significance of spiritual care for nursing.

Additionally, although it would not be possible to alter the nurse's life experience and unethical to attempt to change her beliefs, it may be possible to maximise her awareness of patients' spiritual needs and her ability and confidence in giving systematic spiritual care. Furthermore, the fact that all three nurses who had stated in the questionnaire that they had never identified a spiritual need, through discussion at interview became aware of having done so, suggests that it may be possible to teach nurses greater awareness of patients' spiritual needs. This could perhaps be achieved by using self awareness/sensitivity teaching. This was an approach adopted by both Hitchens (1988) and Piles (1986) based on their findings that the most powerful factor determining how nurses gave spiritual care was their personal faith/value system. Furthermore, Forrest (1989) advocates sensitivity teaching in enabling nurses to care. Self awareness/sensitivity teaching could be conducted in small groups where personal patient encounters or fictitious patient scenarios were explored and analysed with the application of the nursing process. Further research would, however, be required to evaluate the effectiveness of these teaching approaches.

Having maximised the potential of the nurse to recognise patients' spiritual needs and give spiritual care, it would appear that there may be some nurses better able to give spiritual care than others. It would be necessary, therefore, to include in any teaching programme the importance of nurses realising their own limitations and knowing when and how to refer with the minimum of disruption to the nursing process.

It may be possible to increase the efficiency of the referral process by employing measures to facilitate the application of the nursing process to spiritual care. For instance, admission sheets could be altered to include a spiritual assessment and care plans adapted to include space for planning, implementing and evaluating spiritual care. In order to facilitate collaboration between nurses and clergy, it may be beneficial for nurses to: keep a list of the clergy's telephone numbers and 'on-call' times; communicate more with the clergy and discuss certain patients with them as they enter and leave the ward; include the clergy in ward planning/patient profile discussions so that he is treated as a valued member of the health care team. Given the workload of the clergy, the extent of his involvement may, however, be limited.

The findings indicate that even if the nurse's ability to give spiritual care was maximised and the referral process made more efficient that it may still be difficult for nurses to identify the spiritual needs of patients belonging to 'high risk' groups i.e., those with difficulty in communicating for whatever reason. In some instances patients may simply require more time to enable them to communicate their needs and to be understood. For others, e.g., the institutionalised, it may be beneficial to attempt to unlock their true self or spirit through creative and interactive therapies such as occupational, reminiscence, art and music therapies, as suggested by Charatan (1991). In all cases collaboration with the patient's family/friends may be indicated in order to ascertain what gave them meaning and hope in their lives prior to deterioration in their condition.

In addition, the nurse may be further hindered from giving spiritual care by the ward environment which may have implications for administrative decisions.

Given the influence of the spiritual dimension on the physical realm, perhaps it would be more economically viable in the long term to ensure that staff had enough time to spend with patients to attend to their spiritual needs. This may involve ensuring adequate staffing levels are maintained, for example by employing bank/agency nurses if permanent staff are off sick and altering shift patterns to increase rather than reduce staff overlap and/or including the

182

patient's own minister. The result may be production of a higher patient turn over in wards where cure is the desired goal and reduction in demands on staff e.g., by the 'demanding' patient in wards where care, as opposed to cure, is the main objective. Greater work efficiency and utilisation of resources may, therefore, be outcomes. In such wards it may be possible for time to be set aside as part of the ward routine in order to 'be with' rather than 'do for' the patient. In these wards adequate staff overlap may be particularly important.

Moreover, it may be possible to 'promote' a quiet, peaceful and private 'environment in which the...spiritual beliefs of the individual are respected' (ICN 1973, Part 1) by: having a rest hour as part of the ward routine; having set visiting rather than open visiting; ensuring hospital provision of a chapel or reading/quiet room with no television. Where bed bound patients could not utilise the latter, their beds could be screened to provide privacy.

In conclusion, it would appear that for spiritual care to be given well, many factors require to be present and in the right way. Even in the ideal situation where all the ingredients are present for spiritual care to be given at its best i.e., the nurse with the desired qualities and an environment conducive to spiritual care is provided, there is no guarantee that patients' spiritual needs will be fully met. Perhaps this is because the spirit is not bound to conform to natural laws as the body is. To expect it to do so would be to deny its very nature.

Nightingale (in Henderson and Nite, 1978, p.15) said that nursing's function is:

to put the patient in the best condition for nature to act upon him

The function of the nurse in spiritual care could be considered to involve putting the patient in the best condition for the spiritual realm to act upon him. Perhaps as nurses we can do no more but, it could be argued, no less than this. Clearly further research is required to provide nurses with the necessary guidelines to enable them to function in this way and in so doing enable them to fulfil their obligation to:

promote spiritual health and alleviate spiritual suffering (ICN, 1973)

assist the individual to perform those activities contributing to spiritual health that they would have performed unaided had they been able (Henderson, 1977).

21 Suggestions for further research

One of the limitations of the study noted in this chapter was the inability to generalise the study findings. It would be appropriate, therefore, to replicate the study in other areas of care outwith care of the elderly to see if nurses working in these settings viewed spiritual care similarly or differently to nurses in this study.

The factors identified which appeared to influence the spiritual care nurses in this study gave were merely tentative, therefore, further research would be required to explore this. If the findings were similar this could highlight ways in which excellence in spiritual care could be promoted and, therefore, patients helped to attain an optimum level of well-being, which is the ultimate goal of nursing.

In addition to looking at the nurse's perspective, it would also be appropriate to determine, in care of the elderly and other settings, what patients considered their spiritual needs to be and how they felt they could best be helped to meet these needs. This information would help in the planning of appropriate spiritual care. Studies which looked at both the nurse's and patient's perspectives would indicate the extent to which nurses identify and respond to patients' spiritual needs. Such studies may, therefore, highlight any areas nurses had difficulty in dealing with and thus where further instruction might be indicated. Such combined studies might also go some way to establishing a generally agreed definition of spiritual need and indicators of spiritual distress and spiritual well-being, all of which, according to the literature reviewed, were lacking (Parts 1 and 2).

As highlighted in Part 2, this information would assist in facilitating the giving of spiritual care using the nursing process. A number of possible factors were, however, identified which appeared to interfere with the giving of spiritual care in this way. Further research would be beneficial to identify, more reliably, factors contributing to the fragmentation of care and would, thereby, highlight ways in which continuity of spiritual care could be promoted.

Based on a small sample of nurses it seemed that spiritual care was not included or recorded in patients' care plans, however, further research would be necessary to investigate this in a larger sample. Attention could then focus on exploring ways in which spiritual care could best be incorporated into patients' care plans and hence spiritual care be given systematically.

It emerged from the literature review (Part 1), this (Part 4,) and other studies (Part 1), that religious needs were an important aspect of spiritual care. If found to be the case in future research, it may be beneficial to explore hospitals' provision for patients' religious needs.

Finally the literature review highlighted that spiritual care is expected of nurses and should be taught (Part 1). However, from interviewing a small sample of nurses and corresponding with educational establishments, it did not appear that spiritual care was taught to any great extent or in any structured way. Additional research could be undertaken on a larger scale to ascertain if and how spiritual care is currently taught to nurses and then to determine how it could best be taught.

22 Concluding remarks

Returning to the initial aims of the study the author has described how nurses perceived spiritual need and spiritual care and how they reported to have given this care. In addition, factors which appeared to influence the spiritual care nurses gave were identified.

In conclusion, the author has learned much from conducting this study and hopes that some of the above suggestions for further research are pursued by others so that the knowledge base for spiritual care proliferates. In doing so it is hoped that nurses will be better equipped to care for the 'spirit' of their patients which is the very essence of life. Patients could, thus, be helped to achieve their optimum state of health, well-being and quality of life and in so doing nursing would have fulfilled its ultimate goal.

References

American Association of Colleges of Nursing. (1986), *Essentials of College and University Education for Professional Nursing*, AACN: Washington.

Antonovsky, A. (1979), *Health, Stress and Coping*, Jossey-Bass: San Francisco.

Autton, N. (1980). 'The Hospital Chaplain', *Nursing (Add-on Journal)*, Vol. 1, pp. 697-99.

Beland, I.L. and Passos, J.Y, (eds.) (1975), *Clinical Nursing: Pathological and Psychosocial Approaches*, MacMillan: New York.

Blythe, P. (1975), *Stress: the Modern Day Sickness*, Pan Books: London.

Bowlby, R. (1980), 'Chaplains are Different',*British Medical Journal*, Vol. 281, pp. 1689.

Brewer, D.C. (1979), 'Life Stages and Spiritual Well-being', in Moberg, D.O. (ed.), *Spiritual Well-being: Sociological Perspectives*, University Press of America: Washington.

Burnard, P. (1989), *Counselling Skills for Health Professionals*, Chapman and Hall: London.

Burns, R.B. (1980), *Essential Psychology*, MTP Press: Lancaster.

Byles, L.S. (1961), *A Survey of Pediatric Hospitals in the United States to Describe the Available Facilities, Personnel, Programs, Policies and Activities Designed to Meet the Spiritual Needs of Hospitalised Children*. Unpublished Master's Thesis: University of Washington.

Carson, V.B. (1989), *Spiritual Dimensions of Nursing Practice*, W.B.Saunders: Philadelphia.

Chadwick, R. (1973), 'Awareness and Preparedness of Nurses to Meet Spiritual Needs', in Fish, S. and Shelly, J.A. *Spiritual Care: the Nurse's Role*, Inter Varsity Press: Illinois.

Chalmers, H.A. (1989). 'Theories and Models of Nursing and the Nursing Process', in Akinsanya, J.A. (ed.)., *Recent Advances in Nursing. Theories and Models of Nursing*, Churchill Livingstone: Edinburgh.

Champion, P.J. and Sear, A.M. (1973), 'Questionnaire Response Rates: a Methodological Analysis', in Cochrane, R. (ed.)., *Advances in Social Research: A Reader*, Constable and Company Ltd: London.

Chance, J.P.L. (1967), *Nurses' Responses to Patients' Spiritual Needs*, Unpublished Master's thesis, Loma Linda University: California.

Chaplin, N.W. (1989), (ed.)., *The Hospital and Health Services Year Book 1989*, The Institute of Health Services Management.

Charatan, F.B. (1991), 'Introducing the 'food of love' into Geriatric Inpatient Units', *Geriatric Medicine*, Vol. 21, pp. 20.

Chomicz, L. (1984), *What are Patients' Spiritual Needs,?* Unpublished B.Sc dissertation, City University: London.

Colliton, M.A. (1981), 'The Spiritual Dimension of Nursing', in Beland, I.L. and Passos, J.Y. (eds.)., *Clinical Nursing: Pathophysiological and Psychosocial Approaches*, Macmillan: New York.

Conrad, N.L. (1985), 'Spiritual Support for the Dying', *Nursing Clinics of North America*, Vol. 20, pp. 415-26.

Cox, T. (1978), *Stress*, Macmillan: London.

DiCaprio, N.S. (1974), *Personality Theories: Guides to Living*. Saunders: Philadelphia.

Dickinson, C. (1975), 'The Search for Spiritual Meaning', *American Journal of Nursing*, Vol. 75, pp. 1789-93.

Dominian, J. (1983), 'Doctor as Prophet', *British Medical Journal*, Vol. 287, pp. 1925-27.

Dubree, M. and Vogelpohl, R. (1980), 'When Hope Dies - So Might the Patient', *American Journal of Nursing*, Vol. 80, pp. 2046-49.

Ferrans, C.E. and Powers, M.J. (1985), 'Quality of Life Index: Development and Psychometric Properties', *Advances in Nursing Science*, Vol. 8, pp. 15-24.

Fish, S. and Shelly, J.A. (1978), *Spiritual Care: The Nurse's Role*, Inter Varsity Press: Illinois.

Fitzpatrick, J.J. and Whall, A.L. (1983), *Conceptual Models of Nursing: Analysis and Application*, Robert. J. Brady: New Jersey.

Flesner, R. (1981), *Development of a Measure to Assess Spiritual Distress in the Responsive Adult*. Unpublished Master's thesis, Marquette University: Milwaukee.

Forcese, D.P. and Richer, S. (1973), *Social Research Methods*, Prentice-Hall: New Jersey.

Forrest, D. (1989), 'The Experience of Caring', *Journal of Advanced Nursing*, Vol.14, pp. 815-23.

Frankl, V.E. (1959), *Man's Search for Meaning*, Washington Square Press: Washington.

Gardner, R. (1983), 'Miracles of Healing in Anglo-Celtic Northumbria as Recorded by the Venerable Bede and his Contemporaries: a Reappraisal in the Light of Twentieth Century Experience'. *British Medical Journal*, Vol. 287, pp. 1927-33.

Goode, W.J. and Hatt, P.K. (1952), *Methods in Social Science Research*, McGraw-Hill: New York.

Gordon, S.E. and Stokes, S.A. (1989), 'Improving Response Rate to Mailed Questionnaires', *Nursing Research*, Vol. 38, pp.375-76.

Granstrom, S.L. (1985), 'Spiritual Nursing Care for Oncology Patients', *Topics in Clinical Nursing*, Vol. 7, pp. 39-45.

Grubb, G. (1977), 'The Pastor's Role in Visiting the Sick', *Nursing Mirror*, Vol. 144, p. 33.

Hamel-Cooke, C.K. and Cope, D.H.P. (1983), 'Not an Alternative Medicine at St.Marlebone Parish Church', *British Medical Journal*, Vol. 287, pp. 1934-36.

Hargreaves, I. (1979), 'Theoretical Considerations', in Kratz, C.R. (ed.)., *The Nursing Process*, Bailliere Tindall: London.

Henderson, V. (1973), 'The Nature of Nursing', In Auld, M.E and Birum, L.H (Compilers)., *The Challenge of Nursing: a Book of Readings*, Mosby.

Henderson, V. (1977), *Basic Principles of Nursing Care*, ICN: Geneva.

Henderson, V. and Nite, G. (eds.) (1978), *Principles and Practice of Nursing*, MacMillan: New York.

Highfield, M. and Cason, C. (1983), 'Spiritual Needs of Patients: are they Recognised?', *Cancer Nursing*, Vol. 6, pp. 187-92.

Hitchens, E.W. (1988), *Stages of faith and values development and their implications for dealing with spiritual care in the student nurse-patient relationship*, Unpublished ED.D thesis, University of Seattle:Seattle.

Hockey, L. (1979), *A study of district nursing The development and progression of a long term research programme*, Unpublished PhD thesis City University: London.

Hoinville, G., Jowell, R. and Associates (1978), *Survey Research Practice*, Heineman: London.

ICN (1973), *Code for Nurses. Ethical Concepts Applied to Nursing*, ICN: Geneva.

ICN (1977), *The Nurse's Dilemma. Ethical Considerations in Nursing Practice*, ICN: Geneva.

Illich, I. (1975), *Medical Nemesis. An Expropriation of Health. Ideas and Progress*, Calder and Boyars: London.

Ironbar, N.O. (1983), *Self Instruction in Psychiatric Nursing*, Bailliere Tindall: London.

Jacik, M. (1989), 'Spiritual Care of the Dying Adult', in Carson, V.B. (ed.)., *Spiritual Dimensions of Nursing Practice*, W.B. Saunders: Philadelphia.

Kane, E. (1985), *Doing Your Own Research*, Marion Boyars: London.

Kealey, C. (1974), *The Patient's Perspective on Spiritual Needs*, Unpublished Master's thesis, University of Missouri: Columbia.

Kiening, M.M. (1978), 'Spiritual Needs of the Psychiatric Patient', in Dunlap, L.C. (ed.)., *Mental Health Concepts Applied to Nursing*. John Wiley; New York.

Kim, M.J., McFarlane, G. and McLane, A. (1984) (eds.), *Classification of Nursing Diagnoses: Proceedings of the Fifth National Conference*. C.V. Mosby: St.Louis.

Kirkpatrick, E.M. (ed.)., (1983), *Chambers 20th Century Dictionary*, W & R Chambers: Edinburgh.

Kramer, P. (1957), *A Survey to Determine the Attitudes and Knowledge of a Selected Group of Professional Nurses Concerning Spiritual Care of the Patient*. Unpublished Master's thesis, University of Oregon: Oregon.

Kratz, C. (1979). (ed.), *The Nursing Process*, Bailliere Tindall: London.

Lecture Notes 101, *The Limits of Medicine*, Queen Margaret College: Edinburgh.

Lewis, J.E. (1957), *A Resource Unit on Spiritual Aspects of Nursing for the Basic Nursing Curriculum of a Selected School of Nursing*, Unpublished Master's thesis, University of Washington: Seattle.

Limandri, B.J. and Boyle, D.W. (1978), 'Instilling Hope', *American Journal of Nursing*, Vol. 78, pp. 79-80.

McClymont, M., Thomas, S. and Denham, M. (1986), *Health Visiting and the Elderly*, Churchill Livingstone: Edinburgh.

MacDonald, A.M. (ed.)., (1972), *Chambers 20th Century Dictionary*, W.R. Chambers, Edinburgh.

McGhee, R.F. (1984), 'Hope: a Factor Influencing Crisis Resolution', *Advances in Nursing Science*, 6, pp. 34-44.

McGilloway,F.A. and Donnelly, L. (1977), 'Religion and Patient Care: the Functionalist Approach', *Journal of Advanced Nursing*, Vol. 2, pp. 3-13.

McGilloway, O. and Myco, F. (eds.), (1985), *Nursing and spiritual care*, Harper & Row: London.

Marriner, A. (1983), *The Nursing Process. A Scientific Approach to Nursing Care*, C.V. Mosby: Missouri.

Martin, C., Burrows, C. and Pomillo, J. (1976), 'Spiritual needs of patients study' in Fish, S and Shelly, J.A. (1978), *Spiritual care: the nurse's role*, Inter Varsity Press: Illinois.

Martin, J.E. and Carlson, C.R. (1988), 'Spiritual Dimensions of Health Psychology' in: Miller, W.R. and Martin, J.E. (eds.)., *Behaviour Therapy and Religion*, Sage Publications: Beverley Hills.

Maslow, A.H. (1970), 'Motivation and Personality' in DiCaprio, N.S. (ed.). (1974), *Personality Theories: Guides to Living*, Saunders: Philadelphia.

Moberg, D. (1979), *Spiritual Well-being: Sociological Perspectives*, University Press of America: Washington.

Moser, C.A. and Kalton, G. (1971), *Survey Methods in Social Investigation*. Heinman: London.

Murray, R. and Zentner, J. (1975), *Nursing Concepts for Health Promotion*, Prentice Hall: New Jersey.

Myco, F. (1985 a), 'Religion, Magic and Medicine as a Response to Spiritual Need: an Historical Overview' in McGilloway, O. and Myco, F. (eds.)., *Nursing and spiritual care*, Harper and Row: London.

Myco, F. (1985 b), 'Prologue' in McGilloway, O. and Myco, F. (eds.)., *Nursing and Spiritual Care*, Harperand Row: London.

Narayanasamy, B. (1991), *Spiritual Care: a Resource Guide*. BKT Information Services & Quay Publishing LTD: Nottingham.

NBS. (1990), *Nursing Education. Preparation for Practice 1992*, July.

Norusis, M.J /SPSS Inc. (1988), *SPSS/PC + V2.0 Base manual for the IBM PC/XT/AT and PS/2*, SPSS Inc.: Chicago.

O'Brien, M. E. (1982), 'Religious Faith and Adjustment to Long-term Haemodialysis', *Journal of Religion and Health*, Vol. 21, p. 68.

O'Neill, J. (1984), *The Use of Nursing Records in the Evaluation of Nursing Care*, Unpublished M.Sc thesis, University of Manchester: Manchester.

Oppenheim, A.N. (1966), *Questionnaire Design and Attitude Measurement*, Heineman: London.

Orenstein, A. and Phillips, W.R. (1978), *Understanding Social Research: an Introduction*, Allyn and Bacon Inc.: Massachusetts.

Patey, E.H. (1963), 'Has Science Made Religion Out of Date?' *Nursing Mirror*, Vol. 115, p. 476.

Patey, E.H. (1977), 'The Sacred and the Secular', *Nursing Mirror*, Vol.145, pp. 25-26.

Peck, M.L. (1981), 'The Therapeutic Effect of Faith', *Nursing Forum*, Vol. 20, pp. 153-166.

Penrose, V. and Barret, S. (1982), 'Spiritual Needs: in Sickness I Lack Myself', *Nursing Mirror*, Vol. 154, pp. 38-9.

Piepgras, R. (1973), 'The other dimension: spiritual health' in Auld, M.E. and Birum, L.H. (eds.), *The challenge of nursing: a book of readings*, Mosby.

Piles, C.L. (1986), *Spiritual Care: Role of Nursing Education and Practice. A Needs Survey for Curriculum Development*. Unpublished PhD thesis, University of Saint Louis: Saint Louis.

Polit, D.F. and Hungler, B.P. (1987), *Nursing Research: Principles and Methods*. J.B. Lippincott Company: Philadelphia.

Rachman, S.J. and Philips, C. (1978), *Psychology and medicine*, Penguin: Hammondsworth.

Reed, J and Bond, S (1991), 'Nurses' Assessment of Elderly Patients in Hospital', *International Journal of Nursing Studies*, Vol. 28, pp. 55-64.

Reid, N.G. and Boore, J.R.P. (1987), *Research Methods and Statistics in Health Care*, Edward Arnold: London.

Renetzky, L. (1979), 'The fourth dimension: applications to the social services', in Moberg, D.O. (ed.), *Spiritual Well-being: Sociological Perspectives*. University Press of America: Washington.

Riehl-Sisca, J. (1989), *Conceptual Models for Nursing Practice*, Appleton and Lange: Connecticut.

Rinear, E.E. and Buys, A.M. (1985), 'Spiritual and Religious Dimensions of Psychiatric Mental Health Nursing', in Burgess, A.W. (ed.)., *Psychiatric Nursing in the Hospital and the Community*. Prentice-Hall: New Jersey.

Robin, S.S. (1973), 'A Procedure for Securing Returns to Mail Questionnaires' in Cochrane, R. (ed.)., *Advances in Social Research: A Reader*, Constable and Company Ltd: London.

Rogers, M. (1970), *An Introduction to the Theoretical Basis of Nursing*, F.A. Davis: Philadelphia.

Roper, N., Logan, W., and Tierney, A. (1985), *The Elements of Nursing*, Churchill Livingstone: Edinburgh.

Ross, L. (nee Waugh), (1994), 'Spiritual Aspects of Nursing', *Journal of Advanced Nursing*, Vol. 19, pp. 439-47.

Ross, L. (nee Waugh), (1995), 'The Spiritual Dimension: Its Importance to Patients' Health, Well-being and Quality of Life and its Implications For Nursing Practice, *International Journal of Nursing Studies*, Vol. 32, pp. 457-68.

Samarel, N. (1991), *Caring For Life and Death*, Hemisphere Publishing Corporation: New York.

Seidel, J., Kjolseth, R. and Seymour, E. (1988), *The Ethnograph. A Program for the Computer Assisted Analysis of Text Based Data*, Qualis Research Associates: Colorado.

Selye, H. (1980), *Selye's Guide to Stress Research*. Vol.1, Van Nostrand Reinhold: New York.

Seligman, M.E.P. (1974), 'Submissive Death: Giving up on Life', *Psychology Today*, Vol. 7, pp. 80-5.

Seligman, M.E.P. (1975), *Helplessness: on Depression, Development and Death*, Freeman: San Francisco.

Shelly, J.A. and John, S.D. (1983), *Spiritual Dimensions of Mental Health*. Inter Varsity Press: Illinois.

Sims, C. (1987), 'Spiritual Care as a Part of Holistic Nursing', *Imprint*, Vol. 34, pp. 63-4, 67.

Simsen, B.J. (1985), *Spiritual Needs and Resources in Illness and Hospitalisation*, Unpublished M.Sc thesis, University of Manchester: Manchester

Stallwood-Hess, J. (1969), 'Spiritual Needs Survey', in Fish, S. and Shelly, J.A.(1978), *Spiritual Care: the Nurse's Role*, InterVarsity Press: Illinois.

Stoll, R.I. (1979), 'Guidelines for Spiritual Assessment', *American Journal of Nursing*, Vol. 79, pp. 1574-7.

Swaim, L. (1962), *Arthritis, Medicine and Spiritual Laws*, Chilton Book Company: Philadelphia.

Tari, M. (1978), *Like a Mighty Wind*, Kingsway: Eastbourne.

Thorson, J.A. and Cook, T.C. (eds.)., (1980), *Spiritual Well-being of the Elderly*, Charles. C. Thomas: Springfield.

Travelbee, J. (1971), *Interpersonal Aspects of Nursing*, F.A. Dans: Philadelphia.

Travelbee, J. (1977), 'Interpersonal Aspects of Nursing', in Yura, H. and Walsh, M. (eds.)., (1982), *Human Needs 2 and the Nursing Process*, Appleton Century Crofts: Norwalk.

Tubesing, D.A. (1979), *Wholistic Health. A Whole Person Approach to Primary Health Care*, Heiman Science Press: New York.

UKCC (1984 a), *Code of Professional Conduct for the Nurse, Midwife and Health Visitor*, UKCC: London.

UKCC (1984 b), *Exercising Accountability. A Framework to Assist Nurses, Midwives and Health Visitors to Consider Ethical Aspects of Professional Practice*, UKCC: London.

UKCC (1986), *Project 2000. A New Preparation for Practice*, UKCC: London..

UKCC (1991), 'Code of Conduct Under Review', *Register*, Vol. 9, p. 6.

Vaillot, M.C. (1970), 'Hope: the Restoration of Being'. *American Journal of Nursing*, Vol. 70, pp. 268, 270-3.

Walsh, J.C. (1990), 'The Three Levels of Nursing Care, *Professional Nurse*, Vol. 5, p. 666.

Warwick, D.P. and Lininger, C.A. (1975), *The Sample Survey: Theory and Practice*, McGraw-Hill Inc.

Waugh, L.A. (1986), *Spiritual Care: the Neglected Dimension?* Unpublished B.A. dissertation, Queen Margaret College: Edinburgh.

Youngman, M.B. (1978), *Designing and Analysing Questionnaires*, Nottingham University School of Education: Nottingham.

Yura, H. and Walsh, M. (eds.). (1982*)*, *Human Needs 2 and the Nursing Process*, Appleton Century Crofts: Norwalk.

Zentner, J. et al., (1979), 'Religious Influences on the Person', in Murray, R.B. and Zentner, J.P. (eds.), *Nursing Concepts for Health Promotion*, Prentice Hall: New Jersey.

Zola, I.K. (1978), 'Medicine as an Institution of Social Control: the Medicalisation of Society, in Tuckett, D and Kaufert, J.M (eds.), (1978), *Basic Readings in Medical Sociology*, Tavistock: London.

Bibliography

Allen, C. (1991), 'The Inner Light', *Nursing Standard*, Vol. 5, pp. 52-3.

Artinian, B.M. (1991), 'The Development of the Intersystem Model', *Journal of Advanced Nursing*, Vol.16, pp. 194-205.

Atkinson, R.L., Atkinson, R.C. and Hilgard, E.R. (1981), *Introduction to Psychology*, Harcourt Brace Jovanovich: New York.

Barnard, D. (1984), 'Illness as a Crisis of Meaning: Psycho-spiritual Agendas in Health Care', *Pastoral Psychology*, Vol. 33, pp. 74-82.

Beeny, J. (1990), 'Spiritual Healing', *Nursing Standard*, Vol. 5, pp. 48-9.

Belcher, A.E., Dettmore, D. and Holzemer, S.P. (1989), 'Spirituality and Sense of Well-being in Persons with AIDS', *Holistic Nursing Practice*, Vol. 3, pp.16-25.

Bennett, A.E., and Ritchie, K (1975), *Questionnaires in Medicine a Guide to Their Design and Use*, Oxford University Press: London.

Birol, L. (1981), 'New Approaches in Nursing Practice', in ICN, (1981), *Health Care of All. A Challenge for Nursing*, ICN: Geneva.

Blattner, B. (1981), *Holistic Nursing*, Prentice-Hall: New Jersey.

Blecke, J.R. (1963), *Development of a Tool for Determining Appropriate Nursing Actions in Meeting Spiritual Needs of Patients in Selected Situations*, Unpublished Master's thesis, University of Washington: Washington.

Booth, L. (1984), 'Aspects of Spirituality in San Pedro Peninsula Hospital', *Alcoholism Treatment Quarterly*, Vol.1, pp. 121-3.

Boutell, K.A. and Bozett, F.W. (1990), 'Nurses' Assessment of Patients' Spirituality: Continuing Education Implications', *Journal of Continuing Education in Nursing*, Vol. 21, pp. 172-6.

Brase, C. and Brase, C. (1991), *Understandable Statistics. Concepts and Methods*, D.C Heath and Co.: Masachusetts.

Brittain, J.N. (1986), 'Theological Foundations for Spiritual Care, *Journal of Religion and Health*, Vol. 25, pp. 107-21.

Brittain, J.N., and Boozer, J. (1987), 'Spiritual Care: Integration into a Collegiate Nursing Curriculum', *Journal of Nursing Education*, Vol. 26, pp. 155-60.

Brocklehurst, J. (1978), 'Aging and Health', in Hobman, D. (ed.), (1978), *The Social Challenge of Aging*, Croom Helm: London.

Brooke, V. (1987), 'The Spiritual Well-being of the Elderly', *Geriatric Nursing*, Vol. 8, pp. 194-9.

Burbank, P.M. (1988), *Meaning in Life Among Older Persons*, Unpublished D.N.Sc. thesis, University of Boston: Boston.

Burkhardt, M.A. (1989), 'Spirituality: an Analysis of the Concept, *Holistic Nursing Practice, 3*, pp. 69-77.

Burnard, P. (1987), 'Spiritual Distress and the Nursing Response: Theoretical Considerations and Counselling Skills', *Journal of Advanced Nursing*, Vol.12, pp. 377-82.

Burnard, P. (1988 a), 'Discussing Spiritual Issues with Clients', *Health Visitor*, Vol. 61, pp. 371-2.

Burnard, P. (1988 b), 'Search for Meaning', *Nursing Times*, Vol. 84, pp. 34-6.

Burnard, P. (1988 c), 'The Spiritual Needs of Atheists and Agnostics', *Professional Nurse*, Vol. 4, pp. 130, 132.

Burnard, P. (1989), *Counselling Skills for Health Professionals*, Chapman and Hall: London.

Byrne, M. (1985), 'A Zest for Life', *Journal of Gerontological Nursing*, Vol. 11, pp. 30-3.

Caine, R.M. (1991), 'Incorporating CARE into Caring for Families in Crisis', *AACN Clinical Issues in Critical Care Nursing*, Vol. 2, pp. 236-41.

Caravaglia, L. (1982) (ed.), *Aging and the Human Condition*, Human Sciences Press: New York.

Carlisle, D. (1990), 'Spiritual Services', *Nursing Times*, Vol. 86, pp. 30-1.

Caudrey, A. (1987), 'The Art of Dying', *New Society*, Vol. 82, pp. 14-16.

Clark, C.C. *et al.* (1991), 'Spirituality: Integral to Quality Care', *Holistic Nursing Practice*, Vol. 5, pp. 67-76.

Clemence, M. (1966), 'Existentialism: a Philosophy of Commitment', *American Journal of Nursing*, Vol. 66, pp. 500-5.

Clifford, C. (1985), 'Helplessness: a Concept Applied to Nursing Practice', *Intensive Care Nursing*, 20 February, pp. 19-24.

Clifford, M. and Gruca, J.A. (1987), 'Facilitating Spiritual Care in the Rehabilitation Setting', *Rehabilitation Nursing*, Vol.12, pp. 331-3.

Cochrane, R.(ed.). (1973), *Advances in Social Research: A Reader*, Constable and Company LTD: London.

Collins, S. and Parker, E. (1983), *An Introduction to Nursing. The Essentials of Nursing*, Macmillan Press: London.

Cowie, A.P. (ed.) (1989), *Oxford Advanced Learner's Dictionary*, Oxford University Press: Oxford.

Crow, R. (1982), 'Frontiers of Nursing in the Twenty First Century: Development of Models and Theories on the Concept of Nursing', *Journal of Advanced Nursing*, Vol. 7, pp 111-6.

Darocy, C. (1979), 'An Overlooked but Important Part of Nursing: Religious Considerations in Patient Care', *Journal of Practical Nursing*, Vol. 29, pp. 18-21, 31.

Davidson, A.W. (1978), 'In Search of Models of Care', *Death Education*, Vol. 2, pp. 145-61.

Davies, G. (1980), 'The Hands of the Healer: Has Faith a Place?', *Journal of Medical Ethics*, Vol. 6, pp.185-9.

Dean, L.R. (1962), 'Aging and Decline of Affect', *Journal of Gerontology*, Vol.17, p. 440.

del Valle, S. (1980), 'Spiritual Care and the Nursing Process', *Australasian Nurses Journal*, 9 June, pp. 12-13.

Dettmore, D. (1984), 'Spiritual Care: Remembering Your Patients' Forgotten Needs, *Nursing (Horsham)*, Vol.14, p. 46.

de-Zoysa, I. et al. (1984), 'Perceptions of Childhood Diarrhoea and Its Treatment in Rural Zimbabwe', *Social Science and Medicine*, Vol.19, pp. 727-734.

Dimeo, E. (1980), 'Nursing: Significance for Spiritual Care', *Journal of Religion and Health*, Vol. 19, pp. 240-5.

Dobratz, M.C. (1990), 'Hospice Nursing's Present Perspective and Future Directives', *Cancer Nursing*, Vol.13, pp. 116-22.

Dombeck, M. and Karl, J. (1987), 'Spiritual Issues in Mental Health Care', *Journal of Religion and Health*, Vol. 26, pp.183-97.

Donley, R. (1991), 'Spiritual Dimensions of Health Care. Nursing's Mission', *Nursing Health Care*, Vol. 12, pp. 178-83.

Dopson, L. (1988/89), 'Spiritual Healing...Hospital of St.John of God', *Nursing Times*, Vol.84, pp. 43-5.

Downe-Wamholdt, B. (1986), 'Determinants of Perceived Life Satisfaction in the Institutionalised Elderly', *Nursing Papers*, Vol.18, pp. 45-55.

Dugan, D.D. (1987), 'Death and Dying: Emotional, Spiritual and Ethical Support for Patients and Families', *Journal of Psychosocial Nursing and Mental Health Services*, Vol. 25, pp.21-9.

Ebrahim, S. (1987), 'Improving Elderly People's Quality of Life-What Does it Mean?', *Geriatric Medicine*, Vol. 17, pp. 11-15.

Ellerhorst-Ryan, J. (1985), 'Selecting an Instrument to Measure Spiritual Distress', *Oncology Nursing Forum*, 12, pp.93-4, 99.

Ellis, D. (1980), 'Whatever Happened to the Spiritual Dimension?', *Canadian Nurse*, Vol. 76, pp. 42-3.

Ellison, C. (1983), 'Spiritual Well-being: Conceptualisation and Measurement', *Journal of Psychological Theology*, Vol. 11, p.330.

Emmer, R. and Browne, P. (1984), 'Program Helps Nurses Develop Spiritual Care Skills...St.Joseph's Hospital, Milwaukee', *Hospital Progress*, Vol. 65, pp. 64-6.

Epperly, J. (1983). 'The Cell and the Celestial: Spiritual Needs of Cancer Patients, *Journal of the Medical Association of Georgia*, Vol. 72, pp. 374-6.

Erickson, E.H. and Erickson, J.M. (1986), *Vital Involvement in Old Age: The Experience of Old Age in Our Time*, W.W. Norton and Company Inc.: New York.

Erickson, R.C. (1987), 'Spirituality and Depth Psychology', *Journal of Religion and Health*, Vol. 26, pp. 198-205.

Ferszt, G.G. and Taylor, P.B. (1988), 'When Your Patient Needs Spiritual Comfort', *Nursing*, Vol. 18, pp.48-9.

Field, P.A. and Morse, J.M. (1985), *Nursing Research. The Application of Qualitative Approaches*, Croom Helm: London.

Forbis, P.A. (1988), 'Meeting Patients' Spiritual Needs: Helping Patients to Fulfil Their Spiritual Needs is Part of the Nursing Process', *Geriatric Nursing: American Journal of Care for the Aging*, Vol. 9, pp.158-9.

Fowler, J.W. (1981), *Stages of Faith: The Psychology of Human Development and the Quest for Meaning*, Harper and Row: San Francisco.

Garrett, G. (1983), *Health Needs of the Elderly*, Macmillan Press: London.

Gray, R.M. and Moberg, D.O. (1977), *The Church and the Older Person*, W.B.Eerdwans Publishing Company: MI.

Gubrium, V. (1974), 'Late life: Communities and Environment Policy', in Moberg, D.O (ed.), *Spiritual Well-being in Late Life*, Charles C Thomas: Illinois.

Gutterman, L. (1990), 'A Day Treatment Program for Persons With AIDS. *American Journal of Occupational Therapy*, Vol. 44, pp.234-7.

Guy, R.F. (1982), 'Religion, Physical Disabilities and Life Satisfaction in Older Age Cohorts', *International Journal of Aging and Human Development*, Vol.15, pp. 225-32.

Hale, F.B., Richmond, D.R. and Kunkel, A.R. (1983), 'Training in Behavioural Sciences for Residents in Family Medicine, *Military Medicine*, Vol.148, pp. 254-5.

Hall, C.M. (1986), 'Crisis as an Opportunity for Spiritual Growth', *Journal of Religion and Health*, Vol. 25, pp. 8-17.

Hamner, M.L. (1990), 'Spiritual Needs: a Forgotten Dimension of Care?', *Journal of Gerontological Nursing*, Vol.16, pp. 3-4.

Hardy, A. (1979), *The Spiritual Nature of Man: a Study of Contemporary Religious Experience*, Clarendon Press: Oxford.

Hariman, J. (1979), ' Case Notes and Hypnotic Techniques: Existential Spiritual Exercises', *Australian Journal of Clinical and Experimental Hypnosis*, Vol. 7, pp. 279-81.

Harris, R. and Harris, S. (1980/81), 'Therapeutic Uses of Oral History Techniques in Medicine', *International Journal of Aging and Human Development*, Vol. 12, pp. 27-34.

Hay, M.W. (1982), 'Principles in Building Spiritual Assessment Tools', *American Journal of Hospital Care*, Vol. 6, pp. 25-31.

Henderson, K.J. (1989), 'Dying, God and Anger: Comforting Through Spiritual Care', *Journal of Psychosocial Nursing and Mental Health Services*, Vol. 27, pp. 17-21, 31-2.

Hendlin, S.J. (1985), 'The Spiritual Emergency Patient: Concept and Example Special issue: Psychotherapy and the Religiously Committed Patient', *Psychotherapy Patient*, Vol.1, pp. 79-88.

Hilton, A. (1987), *Research Awareness. A Programme for Nurses, Midwives and Health Visitors. The Ethnographic Perspective. Module 7*, HMSO: London.

Hubert, M. (1963), 'Spiritual Care for Every Patient', *Journal of Nursing Education*, Vol. 2, pp. 9-11, 29-31.

Huff, D (1973), *How to Lie with Statistics*, Pelican: Middlesex.

Hungelmann, J., Kenkel, R.E. and Klassen, L. (1985), 'Spiritual Well-being in Older Adults: Harmonious Interconnectedness', *Journal of Religion and Health*, Vol. 24, pp. 147-53.

Hungelmann, J. *et al.* (1989), 'Development of the JAREL Spiritual well-being Scale', *Classification of Nursing Diagnoses. Proceedings of the Eighth Conference*, pp..393-98.

Hutchings, D. (1991), 'Spirituality in the Face of Death', *Cancer Nursing*, 87, pp. 30-1.

Hutchison, S. (1986), 'Grounded Theory: the Method', in Munhall, P.L and Oiler C.J. (eds.), (1986), *Nursing Research. A Qualitative Perspective*, Appleton-Century-Crofts: Norwalk.

Ingle, J.R. (1988), *The Business of Caring: the Perspective of Men in Nursing*, D.S.N. dissertation, University of Alabama at Birmingham: Alabama.

ICN (1981), *Health Care for All. Challenge for Nursing*, ICN: Geneva.

Jahoda, M. and Warren, N. (1966). (eds.), *Attitudes*, Penguin: Middlesex.

Jourard, S.M. (1970), 'Suicide: an Invitation to Die', *American Journal of Nursing*, Vol. 70, pp. 269, 273-5.

Kennison, M.M. (1987), 'Faith: an Untapped Health Resource', *Journal of Psychosocial Nursing and Mental Health Services*, Vol. 25, pp. 28-30, 32-3.

Kershaw, B. and Salvage, J. (eds.) (1986), *Models for Nursing,*. John Wiley and Sons: Chichester.

Kilby, Father. (1981), 'Let's Remember the Spiritual and Emotional Needs of the Patient', *Australian Nurses Journal*, Vol. 10, pp. 83-5.

Kirschling, J.M. and Pittman, J.F. (1989), 'Measurement of Spiritual Well-Being: a Hospice Caregiver Sample', *Hospice Journal: Physical, Psychosocial and Pastoral Care of the Dying*, Vol. 5, pp. 1-11.

Knapp, R.G. (1985), *Basic Statistics for Nurses*, John Wiley and Sons: New York.

Kravis, T.C. and Warner, C.G. (eds.), (1983), *Emergency Medicine: a Comprehensive Review*: Aspen: Rockville.

Kuhn, C.C. (1988), 'A Spiritual Inventory of the Medically Ill Patient', *Psychiatric Medicine*, Vol. 6, pp. 87-100.

Kushner, H.S. (1984), 'When Children and Adults Suffer.19th Annual Conference of the Association for the Care of Children's Health', *Children's Health Care*, Vol. 14, pp. 68-75.

Kwon, H.J. (1989), 'Perceptions of Spiritual Nursing Care Nurses and Students', *Kanho Hakhoe Chi*, Vol.19, pp. 233-9.

Labun, E. (1988), 'Spiritual Care: an Element in Nursing Care Planning', *Journal of Advanced Nursing*, Vol.13, pp. 314-20.

Lane, J.A. (1987), 'The Care of the Human Spirit', *Journal of Professional Nursing*, Vol. 3, pp. 332-37.

Larson, R. (1978), 'Thirty Years of Research on the Subjective Well-being of Older Americans', *Journal of Gerontology*, Vol. 33, pp. 109-25.

Lawrence, C. (1987), 'An Integrated Spiritual and Psychological Growth Model in the Treatment of Narcissism', *Journal of Psychology and Theology*, Vol. 15, pp. 205-13.

Lewis, D. (1987), 'Spiritual Exercises: All in Good Faith', *Nursing Times*, Vol. 83, pp. 10-43.

Lieff, J.D. (1982), 'Eight Reasons Why Doctors Fear the Elderly, Chronic Illness and Death, *Journal of Transpersonal Psychology*, Vol.14, pp. 47-60.

Lindzey, G., Hall, C.S. and Thompson, R.F. (1975), *Psychology*, Worth: New York.

MacDonald, B.D. (1966), 'This I Believe...Nursing's Many Meanings', in Auld, M.E. and Birum, L.H. (eds.), (1966*). The Challenge of Nursing: a Book of Readings*, Mosby: St.Louis.

MacInnis, K. (1987), 'Prayers', *American Journal of Nursing*, Vol. 87, p. 1256.

McGlone, M.E. (1990), 'Healing the Spirit', *Holistic Nursing Practice*, Vol. 4, pp. 77-84.

Maggs, C. (1988), 'Religious Roots', *Nursing Times*, Vol. 84, pp.28-30.

Males, J. and Boswell, C. (1990), 'Spiritual Needs of People With Mental Handicap', *Nursing Standard*, Vol. 4, pp. 35-7.

Malcolm, J.C. (1987), 'Creative Spiritual Care For the Elderly', *Journal of Christian Nursing*, Vol. 4, pp. 24-6.

Marriner, A. (1983), *The nursing process. A scientific approach to nursing care*, C.V Mosby: Missouri.

Martin, H.W. and Prange, A.J. (1962), 'Human Adaptation - a Conceptual Approach to Understanding Patients', in Auld, M.E. and Birum, L.H. (eds.), *The Challenge of Nursing: a Book of Readings*, Mosby: St.Louis.

Melia, K.M. (1982), 'Tell it as it is - Qualitative Methodology and Nursing Research: Understanding the Student Nurse's World', *Journal of Advanced Nursing*, Vol. 7, pp. 327-35.

Miller, J.F. (1985), 'Assessment of Loneliness and Spiritual Well-being in Chronically Ill and Healthy Adults', *Journal of Professional Nursing*, Vol. 1, pp. 79-85.

Miller, J.F. and Powers, M. J. (1988), 'Development of an Instrument to Measure Hope, *Nursing Research*, Vol.37, pp. 6-10.

Mindel, C.H and Vaughan, C.E. (1978), 'A Multidimensional Approach to Religiosity and Disengagement', *Journal of Gerontology*, Vol. 33, pp. 103-08.

Morrison, R. (1990), 'Spiritual Health Care and the Nurse, *Nursing Standard*, Vol. 5, pp. 34-5.

Moser, C.A. (1958), *Survey Methods in Social Investigation*, Heineman: London.

Nagai, J.M.G. and Burkhardt, M.A. (1989), 'Spirituality: Cornerstone of Holistic Nursing Practice', *Holistic Nursing Practice*, Vol. 3, pp. 18-26.

Nelson, P.B. (1990), 'Intrinsic/extrinsic Religious Orientation of the Elderly: Relationship to Depression and Self Esteem', *Journal of Gerontological Nursing*, Vol.16, pp. 29-35.

Nowotny, M.L. (1989), 'Assessment of Hope in Patients With Cancer: Development of an Instrument', *Oncology Nurse Forum*, Vol. 16, pp. 57-61.

O'Connor, A.P., Wicker, C.A. and Germino, B.B. (1990), 'Understanding the Cancer Patient's Search for Meaning', *Cancer Nursing*, Vol. 13, pp. 167-75.

O'Connor, P.M. (1986), 'Spiritual Elements of Hospice Care', *Hospice Journal*, Vol. 2, pp. 99-108.

O'Connor, P. (1988), 'The role of Spiritual Care in Hospice Are We Meeting Patients' Needs?', *American Journal of Hospice Care*, Vol. 5, pp. 31-7.

Paunonen, M. and Haggman, L.A. (1990), 'Life Situation of Aged Home Nursing Clients', *Journal of Community Health Nursing*, Vol. 7, pp. 167-78.

Peplau, L and Perlman, D. (eds.) (1982*), Loneliness: a Sourcebook of Current Theory, Research and Therapy,* John Wiley and Sons: New York.

Peterson, E.A. (1985), 'The Physical...the Spiritual...Can You Meet all of Your Patients' Needs?', *Journal of Gerontological Nursing*, Vol.11, pp. 23-7.

Peterson, E.A. and Nelson K (1987), 'How to Meet Your Clients' Spiritual Needs', *Journal of Psychosocial Nursing and Mental Health*, Vol. 25, pp. 34-40.

Pettigrew, J.M. (1988), *A Phenomenological Study of the Nurse's Presence with Persons Experiencing Suffering,* Unpublished PhD thesis, Texas Woman's University: Texas.

Piepgras, R. (1968), 'The Other Dimension: Spiritual Help', *American Journal of Nursing*, Vol. 68, pp. 2610-13.

Piles, C.L. (1990), 'Providing Spiritual Care', *Nurse Educator*, Vol.15, pp. 36-41.

Poletti, R. (1981), 'Development of Models and Theories on the Concept of Nursing', in ICN (Ed.) (1981*), Health care for all. Challenge for Nursing*, ICN:Geneva.

Pressman, P. et al. (1990), 'Religious Belief, Depression and Ambulation Status in Elderly Women With Broken Hips,' *American Journal of Psychiatry*, Vol. 147, pp. 758-60.

Presti, H.L. (1990), 'AIDS: the Spiritual Challenge', *Occupational Therapy in Health Care*, Vol.7, pp. 87-102.

Quinless, F.W. and Nelson, M.A. (1988), 'Development of a Measure of Learned Helplessness', *Nursing Research*, Vol. 37, pp. 11-14.

Reed, D. (1970), 'Social Disengagement in Chronically Ill Patients', *Nursing Research*, Vol.19, pp. 109-15.

Reed, P.G. (1986), 'Religiousness Among Terminally Ill and Healthy Adults', *Research in Nursing and Health*, Vol. 9, pp. 35-41.

Reed, P.G. (1987), 'Spirituality and Well-being in Terminally Ill Hospitalised Adults', *Research in Nursing and Health*, Vol.10, pp. 335-44.

Reichman, W.J. (1961), *Use and Abuse of Statistics,* Penguin: Middlesex.

Reid, W.S. (1976), 'Religious Attitudes in Later Life', *Age Concern Today*, Vol. 17, pp. 29-31.

Rew, L. (1986), 'Exercises For Spiritual Growth', *Journal of Holistic Nursing*, Vol. 4, pp. 20-2.

Rew, L. (1989), 'Intuition: Nursing Knowledge and the Spiritual Dimension of Persons', *Holistic Nursing Practice*, Vol. 3, pp. 56-68.

Robertson, I. (1986), 'Learned Helplessness', *Nursing Times*, Vol.17, pp. 28-30.

Rothberg, J.S. (1973), 'Why Nursing Diagnosis?', in Auld, M.E.and Birum, L.H. (eds.), *The challenge of nursing: a book of readings*, Mosby: St. Louis.

Roy, D.J. (1987), 'The spiritual need of the dying', *Journal of Palliative Care*, Vol. 2, pp. 3-4.

Ryan, J. (1984), 'The neglected crisis', *American Journal of Nursing*, Vol. 84, pp. 1257-58.

Ryden, M.B. (1984), 'Morale and Perceived Control in Institutional Elderly', *Nursing Research*, Vol. 33, pp. 130-36.

Ryden, M.B. (1985), 'Environmental Support for Autonomy in the Institutionalised Elderly', *Research in Nursing and Health*, Vol. 8, pp. 363-71.

Salladay, S.A. and McDonnell, M.M. (1989), 'Spiritual Care, Ethical Choices and Patient Advocacy', *Nursing Clinics of North America*, 24, pp. 543-9.

Schnorr, M.A. (1988), *Spiritual Nursing Care: Theory and Curriculum Development*, ED.D. thesis, Northern Illinois University: Illinois.

Seligman, M.E.P. (1975), *Helplessness. On depression, development and death*, W.H. Freeman and Company: New York.

Shelly, J.A. (1982), 'Spiritual Care...Planting Seeds of Hope', *Critical Care Update*, Vol. 9, pp. 7-17.

Shelton, R.L. (1981), 'The Patient's Need of Faith at Death', *Topics in Clinical Nursing*, Vol. 3, pp. 55-59.

Shipman, M.D. (1972), *The limitations of social research*, Longman: London.

Sims, J. (1990), 'Spiritual Sacrifices', *Nursing Times*, Vol. 86, p. 23.

Simsen, B. (1986), 'The Spiritual Dimension...How Patients Coped', *Nursing Times*, Vol. 82, pp. 41-2.

Simsen, B. (1988), 'Nursing the Spirit...Meeting Patients' Spiritual Needs', *Nursing Times*, Vol. 84, pp. 31, 33.

Sirra, E. (1987), *The Implementation of Systematic Nursing in Selected Hospitals in India: a Chronicle of the Change Process*, Unpublished PhD thesis, University of Edinburgh: Edinburgh.

Smith, J.P. (1989), *Virginia Henderson. The First Ninety Years*, Scutari Press: Middlesex.

Sodestrom,K.E., and Martinson, I.M. (1987), 'Patients' Spiritual Coping Strategies: a Study of Nurse and Patient Perspectives', *Oncology Nursing Forum*, Vol. 14, pp. 41-6.

Soeken, K.L., and Carson, V.J (1986), 'Study Measures Nurses' Attitudes About Providing Spiritual Care', *Health Progress*, Vol. 67, pp. 52-5.

Soeken, K.L., and Carson, V.J. (1987), 'Responding to the Spiritual Needs of the Chronically Ill', *Nursing Clinics of North America*, Vol. 22, pp. 603-11.

Sommer, D.R. (1989), 'The Spiritual Needs of Dying Children', *Issues in Comprehensive Pediatric Nursing*, Vol. 12, pp.225-33.

Spreitzer, E. and Snyder, E. (1974), 'Correlates of Life Satisfaction Among the Aged', *Journal of Gerontology*, Vol. 29, pp. 454-58.

Sprent, P. (1981), *Quick statistics*, Penguin: Middlesex.

Stiles, M.K. (1990), 'The Shining Stranger: Nurse-family Spiritual Relationship', *Cancer Nursing*, Vol.13, pp. 235-45.

Stoll, R. (1983), *Indicators of Life Satisfaction in Persons With Life Threatening Diagnoses and Those With Non-life Threatening Diagnoses*, Unpublished PhD thesis, University of Michigan: Michigan.

Stuart, E.M., Deckro, J.P. and Mandle, C.L. (1989), 'Spirituality in Health and Healing: a Clinical Program', *Holistic Nursing Practice*, Vol. 3, pp. 35-46.

Swaffield, L. (1988), 'Religious Roots...Nursing's Religious Origins', *Nursing Times*, Vol. 84, pp. 28-30.

Swaffield, J. (1986), *An Investigation into Dependency Among the Elderly in Two Long Term Wards in Scotland*, Unpublished M.Sc thesis, University of Edinburgh, Edinburgh.

Thomas, S.A. (1989), 'Spirituality: an Essential Dimension in the Treatment of Hypertension', *Holistic Nursing Practice*, Vol. 3, pp. 47-55.

Thorson, J.A. and Powell, F.C. (1990), 'Meanings of Death and Intrinsic Religiosity', *Journal of Clinical Psychology*, Vol. 46, pp. 379-91.

Twycross, R.G. and Lack, S.A. (1990), *Therapeutics in Terminal Cancer*. Churchill Livingstone: New York.

Uyanga, J. (1979), 'The Characteristics of Patients of Spiritual Healing Homes and Traditional Doctors in South Eastern Nigeria', *Social Science and Medicine*, Vol. 13A, pp. 323-9.

Vaillot, M.C. (1966), 'Existentialism: a Philosophy of Commitment', *American Journal of Nursing*, Vol. 66, pp. 500-05.

Walsh, A (1990), *Statistics for the Social Sciences*, Harper and Row: New York.

Warner-Robbins, R.C.G. and Christiana, N.M. (1989), 'The Spiritual Needs of Persons with AIDS', *Family and Community Health*, Vol.12, pp. 43-51.

Weatherall, J. and Creason, N.S. (1987), 'Validation of the Nursing Diagnosis, Spiritual Distress', *Classification of Nursing Diagnoses. Proceedings of the Seventh Conference*, pp.182-5.

Whall, A.L. (1987), 'Self Esteem and the Mental Health of Older Adults', *Journal of Gerontological Nursing*, Vol. 13, pp. 41-2.

Wile, D.B. (1976), 'Personality Styles and Therapy Styles', *Psychotherapy Theory, Research and Practice*, Vol. 13, pp. 303-7.

Wilkinson, S. (1991), 'Factors Which Influence How Nurses Communicate With Cancer Patients', *Journal of Advanced Nursing*, Vol.16, pp. 577-688.

Williams, J.M.G. et al. (1988), *Cognitive Psychology and Emotional Disorders*, John Wiley and Sons: Chichester.

Wilson, G.D. (ed.) (1973), *The Psychology of Conservatism*, Academic Press: London.

Woolley, N. (1990), 'Nursing Diagnosis: Exploring the Factors Which May Influence the Reasoning Process, *Journal of Advanced Nursing*, Vol. 15, pp. 110-17.

Young, L.S. (1968), 'Needs of the Patient As Seen by the Nurse', in Auld, M.E and Birum, L.H. (eds.), *The Challenge of Nursing: a Book of Readings*, Mosby: St Louis.

Learning Resources